The Vegan Solution

*Why the Vegan Diet Often Fails
and How to Fix It*

Matt Stone

with Chris Randall

A proud presentation of:

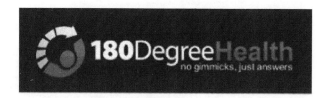

April 2013
ISBN 1484089456
ISBN-13: 978-1484089453

DISCLAIMER

The material provided here is for educational and informational purposes only and is not intended as medical advice. The information contained in this book should not be used to diagnose or treat any illness, metabolic disorder, disease, or health problem. If you have developed a serious illness of some kind, the complexities of dealing with that disorder are best handled by your physician or other professional health care provider, whom you should also consult with before beginning any nutrition or exercise program. Use of the programs, advice, and other information contained in this book is at the sole choice and risk of the reader.

Contents

6

Introduction

What is up with you freakin' vegans? No animal products at all? No butter? No crab legs? No cheebaga cheebaga? A little extreme don't you think – to go all or nothing like that?

If you have a problem with the lack of morality in our modern meat production facilities, or are concerned about environmental degradation of eating higher up on the food chain, or hormones in meat and milk, or whatever – why not just eat less? Why none, zilch, nada?

I mean, I think modern humans abuse electricity and fossil fuels. That doesn't mean I refuse to climb into an automobile or write all my books on legal pads instead of an electricity-guzzling laptop. I drive a car that gets better gas mileage and keep my thermostat off unless it's below 55 or above 80. A 40% reduction in usage is significant. It doesn't have to be 100%.

Would it kill you to have a slice of cheese every now and then? It's not immoral or harmful to your spiritual quest. It will get you closer to God actually. Cheese is fucking Christ!

I kid.

Hi, I'm Matt Stone, independent health researcher and author of way too many health books. I'm just messing with you vegans. Sort of. Hey, if I'm going to write this book which will, WITHOUT A DOUBT, help many of you that read this, at least I can take a few shots and have a little fun. Right?

Guys?

You still reading this?

Okay okay. I don't want to get too carried away. Just know that there may be some playful ribbing of you vegans reading this. It's all in good fun and I truly mean absolutely no harm by it. Just trying to make you smile a little. If you're on a vegan diet and failing enough to purchase this book, I'm sure you could use a smile.

I am not vegan, although I have dabbled with it and countless other diets (none of which I regret from a research perspective, all of which I regret from a personal health perspective). I am a health researcher, and, while I may be a jokester with an odd writing style for a subject as serious as your health and well-being, I assure you that this book is no joke. The things that I discuss are real and absolutely of great importance, and few understand some of the basics of our physiology and the way those basics interact with our food, beverages, and lifestyle the way I do. That's why I have taken it upon myself to write this book. I can help. Therefore I will.

Also, I want to say first and foremost that my self-proclaimed mission is to research human health. If cannibalism was the answer to health I would report on it honestly. If eating babies was the true way to avoid heart disease, I would report on it honestly. If the blood of virgins… Okay you get the point. In other words, the information in this book is in no way about morality, or environmental sustainability, or spiritual enlightenment, or anything other than health. I have my own thoughts about such matters, but that will not interfere in any way with what I've been led to believe is the truth. Thought you should know that in case your mind starts to churn out little "buts" while reading this.

We live in a strange eating world. Just an hour ago my girlfriend showed me an article about the discovery of large amounts of arsenic in chicken. She became freaked out. I told her we had some chicken in the fridge. "Do you want me to fry you up some chicken honey?"

She declined. I suggested we save it for her 7-year old daughter tomorrow. She got even more freaked out.

I told her not to get too upset about it, that there was negative and frightening information about literally every single known food. She began quizzing me about certain foods, challenging me to come up with something harmful or "toxic" about each one of them. It was kind of like the scene in *City Slickers* where the Ben and Jerry's guys have to say the perfect ice cream flavor to accompany sea bass, potatoes au gratin, and asparagus.

http://www.youtube.com/watch?v=4pbVxyL-OeM

The pressure was on.

She asked me about potatoes.

Jackpot! We looked at forums about salicylate sensitivity and all the nasty health problems people experience when they eat foods rich in salicylates like potatoes. Then we went on to look at acrylamide – perfect as we had eaten a few French fries earlier and acrylamide forms when starchy foods like potatoes are fried at high temperatures. Woof!

We went on to look at lectins in other foods most people consider healthy, the dangers of excess beta carotene when she asked me about carrots, and the negative effects that some with SIBO might experience when eating bananas due to all the fructooligosaccharides in 'em. This is to speak nothing of the incredible toxicity of aflatoxin in peanut butter – the food with the highest known ratio of omega 6 to omega 3 fatty acids. Woof!

It was a real blast. You can see why she loves me right? I'm utterly irresistible in the gym shorts I'm wearing for the third day in a row. I think the neighbors can smell my balls through the walls. Hey, that rhymes.

The point is that a lot of really scary and negative information is only a click away.

Likewise, we could have gone through and found the virtues of chicken, the fantastic amount of vitamin E in peanut butter, heard Kevin Gianni and David Infomercial Wolfe talk about the incredible health of some Peruvian villagers deriving 90% of their nutrition from potatoes, and more. We could have built a strong case for or against pretty much all foods if given enough time to thoroughly research a side. No really. You should try it sometime. It's easy.

I bring all this up, not just to make a ball joke (they are timeless though!), but to make you aware of something right off the bat…

There are opposing viewpoints out there and they are all valid in their own skewed way. But if you bury your head in one philosophy and one philosophy only for a long enough period of time, you will get more or less brainwashed by it. With enough exposure to anything, and no contradictory evidence to go with it, just about anything starts to make sense. Plus, you'll feel an ever-increasing sense of pride and communion the more like-minded people you run across. Hell, you might even start shouting these great health discoveries from the rooftops, taking great pride in the gift of immortality you are giving to humanity.

Hey, how ya think I got into this health crap? What, you think I started a blog to pass the time? I just ran out of hiking trails and Maui beaches and cute asses to chase? No way man. It was to save the world with the breakthrough health discoveries I found while researching stuff in books and on the internet. You know, a bunch of stuff that was going to save the world in 2008 but turned out to be wrong and stupid, naïve and incomplete a few years later.

If you have read a bunch of vegan books, hung out with a bunch of vegans, watched *Forks Over Knives* 46 times, know Durianrider's first name, and can pin Ocean and Rip to their vegan biological fathers – you're in trouble sister. The true test is if you know who Gabriel Cousens is and you're able to listen to him speak with a straight face. If you can, I'm here to help you dirty up your brain. That shit has been washed clean. Howie Mandel would eat off that thing it's been so thoroughly powerwashed and disinfected of any biological life.

I'm not saying you have to choose McDonald's over McDougall's (ooh, good title for a Morgan Spurlock documentary!), or jump on a caveman diet. But I do want you to think outside the box a little. I will challenge you a little bit. Not too much. Just a little.

Don't be scared or put the book down, afraid that I will tempt you into the heart of darkness with Double Cheeseburgers disguised as Bocas. I know your identity is tied to your diet. I understand how fragile of a topic this is.

You know what, I'm just gonna go ahead and say it.

A vegan, or at least primarily vegetarian diet has some great health advantages. At least in theory it does. This book is not about ditching it. You do what you want to do. While I will give you a little opposing information to do the aforementioned brain-dirtying a tad, what I want to do in this book is not help you "fix" your vegan diet by becoming a seal-clubbing Eskimo. Rather, I want to help you fix your vegan diet by helping you to design it better, learn some things about your body you never knew before, and potentially help you to clear up some problems you may be experiencing on a vegan diet. While remaining vegan. If you want.

A vegan diet can be many things. Vegan diets are as diverse, if not more diverse, than regular diets all around the globe. This book will be about learning just a few simple basics of how to make your diet fit YOU, instead of you constantly trying to make you fit one of the versions of the vegan diet. No matter who you are or what diet you're on, these rules apply. Vegan or not. Like a good night's sleep, some meditation, or some physical activity out in the sun – there are many things that apply to our physiology that are completely agnostic to any dietary religion. It's these things that I want to bring to your attention.

Overview of the Situation

Warning – you are about to read a TON of generalization. But just about everyone should be able to relate to this scenario. Whether this is how you went on to develop problems on a vegan or near-vegan diet or not, there is still some important lessons to be learned. This will hopefully put together a little foundation for where we are later headed.

At first, a person gets a spark to become vegetarian. Maybe it's a book. For me it was *The Food Revolution* by John Robbins. Maybe a friend that is healthier-looking than you is vegetarian and you think you'll be like that too if you eat the same way. Maybe you start dating a girl that is vegetarian, and you become self-conscious about your meat-eating enough to just throw in the towel and ditch the animal products. Maybe it was a documentary or some other propaganda. Maybe it just felt cool to do something different. Rebel against the way of life you were brought up in. Maybe you had a health problem and sought out answers in books and on the internet – finding passionate people and powerful testimonials swearing that a vegan diet was the answer to your problem(s). I don't know what prompted you to become vegetarian, but it was something.

And it may have started really gently. No official declarations of "I'm Vegan!" Perhaps it started with something much simpler, like "I don't eat red meat anymore," later evolving into deeper and deeper grades of dietary Holiness.

But odds are it was an escalation process of some kind that started with one or a small handful of events. The important thing I want to focus on is the escalation process, and the general sequence of events that takes place for many who have stayed on a vegan diet long enough to develop real health problems that they didn't have prior.

First step is of course the initial spark to pursue vegetarianism, with varying degrees of initial extremism.

Next, those with a perfectionist mindset will start placing increasingly stringent controls on what they eat. It starts with avoiding animal products. Then everything must be organic. Then cooked foods become "dead, devitalized foods" that you don't eat anymore. Then you start choking down 2 pounds of greens per day. When that doesn't work, or you don't feel well from it, the cleanses, fasts, and detoxes begin.

It's this escalation process that represents a general movement in the wrong, not the right, direction.

What happens is that the single-most important nutrient that we derive from food is completely forgotten and left behind. That is the CALORIE. The primary reason we eat is to obtain energy. If we do not obtain sufficient energy from the food we eat, the body compensates for this by lowering metabolic rate. When metabolic rate drops, virtually every system in the human body starts to function poorly.

The next most important thing that we derive from food is the macronutrients – protein, carbohydrates, and fat. These too are completely forgotten by many vegetarians on an obsessive quest for dietary purity, "getting out the toxins" and other pseudo-scientific (okay, non-scientific) pursuits. Getting an insufficient amount of fiber, vitamins, minerals – all that kind of thing may be a problem. But it's a very minor problem compared to getting insufficient amounts of the macronutrients and overall calories. From this point forward, we will call the basic constituents of food needed for immediate proper functioning – those calories and macronutrients, as "The Primary Nutrients."

If you get one thing out of this book, it is to obey the laws of physiology first and foremost. A $500,000 car will not drive if there is no fuel in the tank. You should, ESPECIALLY as a vegan on a restricted diet that excludes so many rich sources of the Primary Nutrients, pay particular attention to what is primary.

But the typical vegan (not that this is just a vegan problem, this problem is seen everywhere in the world of "healthy" diets) has what is primary and what is secondary totally bass ackwards. The problems from having these priorities out of order sneak up in a very subtle and covert way, manifesting in a few pesky problems like dry hair, more bloating after eating a meal, reduced sex drive, and cold feet – just to name a few common ones. A few early signs. Unfortunately one of two things usually happens at this point...

1. The diet is presumed to be perfect, and other treatments are sought after – like removing mercury fillings, food allergy testing, taking supplements, doing a fast, getting energy treatments, acupuncture, colonics, and so forth to infinity
2. Or the diet gets even tighter and more strict as the health problems emerging are presumed by the person to be from lack of adherence to the diet, not caused by the diet itself, which is more likely

Both of these routes lead to increased paranoia, lots of unnecessary expenditures on empty cures and remedies, even more puritanical health food diet adherence, more damage, and the digging of an ever-deeper hole. This speaks nothing of the social isolation that often occurs in tandem with this escalation process.

All the while the primary nutrients, the things our bodies need the most to carry out proper function and maintain a healthy metabolism and all the functions related to it (sex, digestion, sleep, mood stability, wound healing, blood sugar regulation, and others), drift farther and farther out of mind.

This is the process that you, as an individual who is suffering many health problems on a vegan diet, probably need to reverse. And that will be the subject of this book, basically.

I originally became inspired to write this book because of my expertise of the many ways in which a lack of adequate calorie intake – starvation basically – manifests. Some of the common negatives that vegans often experience such as hair loss, loss of sex drive or menstruation, feeling freezing cold, low energy, anemia, severe gas and bloating, emotional instability – can all be attributable to starvation or the low metabolism that accompanies undernutrition.

Many assume that these problems are from lack of animal products in the diet. I certainly figured that in the past. Sometimes it probably is. Many times it isn't. I suspect from people who I have dealt with that most problems on a vegan diet are actually NOT from a massive deficiency of some animal-sourced vitamin, protein, or otherwise. I think many people are just freaking starving and may also be suffering the metabolic consequences of losing body fat – something everyone presumes is healthy but in scientific study is thought to typically cause more or less permanent metabolism suppression until body fat levels are adequately replenished.

Identifying such a problem and taking simple action steps to correct the problem is what this very simple but powerful book is about. Let's get on with it already.

Starvation

Not doing so "hot" on a vegan diet? I propose that you are starving – meaning that you simply are not, and haven't been for quite some time, consuming enough calories for your body to work like it should. Before we dig any deeper, here are some of the symptoms of inadequate food intake that were so eloquently documented in the most thorough investigation on the subject – *The Biology of Human Starvation* by Ancel Keys.

During World War II, Ancel Keys rounded up a bunch of male volunteers for extensive study of the effects of calorie deprivation. While most think that 1500-calories is an adequate amount of calories, it most certainly wasn't for the men, 150-ish pounds on average at the start of the experiment. This was plenty low to cause substantial weight loss, a dramatic lowering of the metabolic rate, and all the dysfunction that ensues when metabolic rate slows dramatically. The men were eating more than twice that amount on a typical day prior to the start of the experiment.

Here are some of the basic things they experienced…

"A continuous gnawing sensation in the stomach"

"Almost impossible to keep warm, even with an excessive amount of clothing."

"They also experienced a 40% decrease in metabolism."

"The men also experienced significant decreases in blood pressure and pulse rate; they suffered from anemia, the inability to concentrate, and marked weakness during physical activity."

"They also experienced 'a decrease in sexual interest and expression, which, according to some of the men, reached the point of obliteration.'"

"[Afterwards], the men 'almost invariably over-ate…In particular, the cravings for "sweets and accessory foods of all kinds,' — i.e., snacks were now free to be indulged, and so they were.'"

"Benedict's young subjects managed to regain all the lost weight and body fat in less than twelve weeks."

"Food quickly became the subject of conversation and daydreams. The men compulsively collected recipes and studied cookbooks. They chewed gum and drank coffee and water to excess; they watered down their soups to make them last."

"Eventually, five of the subjects succumbed to what Keys and his colleagues called 'character neurosis…' it 'bordered on psychosis…' One subject…broke down 'weeping [with] talk of suicide and threats of violence,' and was committed to the psychiatric ward at the University Hospital."

I've personally experienced the same degree of starvation so I can attest to all of the above-mentioned tendencies. There is overlap of course between these symptoms and the symptoms those with eating disorders experience – or even just regular "dieters" that are purposefully restricting their diet significantly. They also go hand in hand with those who suffer from hypothyroidism, as a reduced metabolic rate is at the root of many conditions.

There are countless others. I toyed with the idea of posting my entire collection of quotes from the *Biology of Human Starvation* just to show the many connections. But even that is just scratching the surface. Author

Mark Starr in his book about hypothyroidism throws down with a chapter called "Symptoms" that is 85-pages long. Anything and everything is likely to function suboptimally when the energy supply in your cells is low. There can be many root causes, but certainly a low-calorie diet is the most surefire way to achieve it.

Other common things that you might experience that come to mind are...

1. Thinning hair, dry hair, or hair loss
2. Slow fingernail growth or cracked, brittle fingernails
3. Dry skin, especially around the hands and lower legs and feet
4. Thinning eyebrows
5. Slow-growing leg hair, beard, other shaved areas, or loss of body hair
6. Loss of menstrual cycle or more severe PMS or other irregularities
7. PCOS
8. Infertility, miscarriage, pregnancy complications, poor lactation
9. Constipation
10. Bloating or delayed stomach emptying
11. Irritable bowel syndrome and/or small intestine bacterial overgrowth (SIBO)
12. Heartburn, indigestion, nausea after eating
13. Dry mouth

14. Excessive thirst
15. Frequent urination, nighttime urination, strong sudden urges to urinate
16. Belly fat, especially with low muscle mass/poor strength
17. Puffy eyes
18. Water retention
19. Low platelets
20. Low red blood cell counts
21. Low white cell counts
22. Low sperm counts, poor sperm motility
23. Reduced size of testes
24. Low testosterone
25. Low progesterone
26. Adrenal fatigue
27. Tooth decay, sensitive teeth
28. Anxiety
29. Depression
30. Insomnia

Again, this is still scratching the surface of all the systems that are affected by a reduced metabolic rate, but it's a good start. These are some of the more common manifestations.

Of course, many vegans experience several of these problems. And, before you get your hemp undies in a wad, I would like to remind you that many people on many diets experience a suppressed metabolism. Even that Dr. Atkins guy (I think you vegans call him Satan, or is that Seitan?) knew that there were infinite dietary paths to inducing a low metabolism.

"Remember that prolonged dieting ([low-carb]*, low-fat, low-calorie, or a combination) tends to shut down thyroid function."*

It's not a problem exclusive to veganism by any means. In fact, when I wrote a book bashing the Paleo diet (*12 Paleo Myths*) I mentioned basically the exact same "symptoms" of the Paleo diet failing miserably. Here are the symptoms I listed in that book, this again being a very abbreviated list. Many of the items below strongly overlap with the negatives many vegans experience, as any restricted diet frequently results in a downregulated metabolism. There are infinite paths to the same destination…

1. Cold Hands and Feet
2. Wiener Malfunction
3. Reduced Sex Drive
4. Loss of Menstruation
5. Infertility
6. Frequent Urination/Polyuria
7. Night Sweats
8. Anxiety
9. Irritability
10. Waking at 4am/Insomnia

11. Lightheadedness
12. Constipation
13. Gastroparesis/Delayed Stomach Emptying
14. Acid Reflux
15. High LDL cholesterol
16. Low testosterone
17. Puffy Eyes/Water Retention
18. Autoimmune disease
19. Increased Allergies/Sensitivities
20. Hypoglycemia

The good news is that most of the items on the two lists I've given you are pretty easily-correctable with the right approach.

You just have to like, totally cleanse! Juice feasting on kale juice will give you all the nutrients you need. Our bodies don't even need calories to function anyhow. Robert O. Young says we run off of electrons. Just alkalize and you will feel great and test the limits of the maximum human lifespan!

Uh, no.

From Fat to Fit – Chris Randall's Story

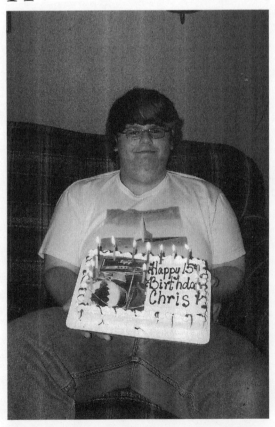

Hey there. My name's Chris Randall. If you don't know who I am, I'm this crazy dude on the Internet who makes all sorts of videos and stuff on the topic of health, nutrition, and weight loss. Well, one of the many who do so. I used to weigh well over 320lbs. during my childhood, but have since lost around 150lbs. of fat by changing up my diet. Oh yeah, I'm also a Vegan.

Yep, that's right:

Vegan with a capital V. I'm not a VEGAN!!! however, mind you. I won't throw red paint on your fur coat as you walk by and call you a murderer. Heck, even if we go out for dinner together and I have baked potatoes with veggies and salad and you order a big, bloody steak, I won't even refer to you as a corpse-crunching lunatic and ask you, "How do you like your vulture food?" Nobody likes that, and that never changed anyone's mind or inspired anyone.

Oh, and if I was stranded on an island with the option of eating a steak or getting shot in the head, I'd probably just take the bullet. Hypothetical questions stress me out.

Glad we cleared those things up.

But I do personally feel very strongly about everything that Veganism entails. And not just so I can be a part of the club and show up and drink the Kool-Aid (the green batch that Durianrider makes is my favorite). It really means a lot to me. I know, I know. I could have a few slices of cheese or some oysters every now and again and not drop dead of a heart attack the next hour or get bowel cancer. It honestly just doesn't jive with me, and that's why I do what I do.

I know that there are thousands of people out there just like me who are in the same position I am. You're passionate about a vegan diet and lifestyle and you want to maintain that and be the best person you can be. But maybe you're worried because that one guy or gal who was vegan for a while started experiencing some issues on their vegan diet. They went back to eating fish heads and grass-fed butter and everything magically got better again.

For me, I have never really experienced any issues on my vegan diet, or at least what I saw as obvious issues. I went from a Standard American Diet when I was about 15 years old to a starch-based, McDougall-style diet with lots of rice, potatoes, corn, pasta, etc. I maintained that for about 1 ½-2 years and felt fantastic. The weight started pouring off and everything was going perfectly.

When I was about 17 years old, I stumbled upon the notion of a Raw Food Diet. Yeah, I went through a serious green-juicing, nut-butter-laden, super-food-stoked phase. Shortly after that, I found out about the high-fruit raw vegan diet, also commonly

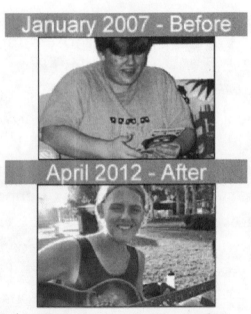

January 2007 - Before

April 2012 - After

referred to as, "The 80/10/10 Diet": Basically, a diet high in carbs, low in fat, with raw fruit being the primary source of calories. 30 Bananas A Day ring a bell?

I did really well with everything and certainly didn't have all my teeth fall out of my face or anything else scary that some people might say would happen. The only real downside that I could see is that I was definitely cold frequently. In my home of southeastern South Dakota, USA, the winters are relentless. Cold, wind, and ice is the name of the game November-March every year. Long pants, thick socks, and long sleeve shirts were a must. Bedtime usually meant an electric blanket and a space heater too. Makes me chilly just thinking about it!

I've come a long way since then. Now, even in the dead of winter, I sleep in a thin pair of boxer shorts (at most) and only sometimes with a thin blanket. A few months ago I was even walking around Aspen, Colorado (you know, where the beer flows like wine?) in my shorts in the middle of December. It's pretty cold there too.

So why, might you ask, is a vegan contributing to a book on the topic of diet and nutrition, written by someone who's not a vegan or doesn't inherently promote a vegan diet?

Because I want to see people succeed and be happy and healthy on a vegan lifestyle. That's what I'm passionate about. I'm open enough to listen to anyone's perspective and see if I can form a sounder stance as a result. I've seen more than my fair share of shivering, somewhat neurotic, hungry fellow vegans trying to live off of green juice, almonds, and Goji berries. When they start experiencing symptoms, they insist that they need to do more cleansing and become even purer. So they cut more foods out of their diet, become stricter and more obsessive, and ultimately just hit rock bottom. This is what I coined the "Paleo Advocate, Vegan-Basher Maker Equation." It goes like this: vegan diet + bad information – caloric density = crash and burn. Or something like that. I was never very good at math.

Heck, raw beef liver would start looking good to me too if I let myself get that hungry! One of my Paleo buddies actually admitted to me just the other day that while he was at the post office shipping off a copy of Gary Taubes's *Why We Get Fat* to his father, the packing peanuts started to look appetizing. Maybe he needs more carbs.

Of course, this isn't inherent to a vegan diet at all, it could happen on any diet. Some people promoting a vegan diet just happen to get a little too caught up in specific nutrients and nutrient-density and forget about the biggest reason we eat food: calories.

No, I honestly don't believe any issues that any vegan might experience on their diet is at all related to lack of animal products. It's simply basic, physiologic needs that possibly aren't being met. So if you're a bit chillier than you'd like to be or your hair's not growing as fast as you'd like, leave that organic butter on the shelf for just a moment and hear us out.

Metabolism

I don't give a flying rat's ass what you eat. All that matters to me is that your "machine" is functioning correctly.

Another way to phrase this is "You are not what you eat, you are what your body does with what you eat."

Still not getting it?

I've also said over the years that "People should stop focusing so much on nutrition and start focusing on how their bodies work."

Really confused now? I'll see if I can bring it home with this one...

Steer your efforts away from the small details of your diet, and redirect them towards getting the systems of your body working correctly.

At the root of proper function is the metabolism, which starts with energy production by the mitochondria in your cells and extends into virtually every system of the body – reproductive, digestive, hormonal, osmoregulatory, and so on. It's these systems that you should be seeking to improve. Improvement in metabolism yields improvement in the function of any or many of these systems, and that represents a powerful increase in overall health. Get the systems of the body working better and any number of health improvements can take place, including, in some fortunate cases, improvement or reversal of some pretty nasty ailments and diseases.

Although some general rules apply, for the most part the diet and lifestyle changes required to improve metabolism at any given point in time are highly individual. They also depend on the circumstances – they are not static. For example if you have developed a low metabolism on a low-fat diet, fat might be the single most therapeutic agent in restoring normal metabolic function. If you've been sitting around doing absolutely no physical activity, exercise might play a role in restoring proper energy production, whereas in an over-trained athlete some hardcore couchriding in lieu of physical activity is a must. And so on.

If you direct your attention towards how your body is functioning, and look closely at how your body responds to certain things metabolically, then you can fine-tune this kind of thing. There is nothing in the "health game" like some well-informed self-assessment. Nothing. It outperforms just about every diet, menu plan, exercise program, supplement, and alternative health intervention out there.

Without going into exhaustive and painstaking detail to reassure you of the validity of the following as metabolism indicators, I'll jump right to a decent list of markers that you can use as sort of a metabolic scorecard. The objective is to achieve competency or excellence in ALL of the following categories. I think you'll agree and soon come to understand how powerful some of these simple things can be when you start making some improvements.

Metabolism Scorecard

1.   Your waking oral/rectal/vaginal body temperature should be at least 98 degrees F/36.7 C every day – higher temps are even better.
2.   Your body temperature should rise even higher after meals and during the day.
3.   Your hands and feet should feel warm most of the time at normal room temperature.
4.   You should experience a feeling of radiating plentiful body heat in general – dressing lighter and feeling as warm or warmer than those around you.
5.   You should have fast-growing hair (head and body) and fingernails, with good shine to the hair and hardness to the nails.

6.   You should have at least one, hopefully more, large bowel movements per day that do not require straining or the use of laxatives, magnesium overdosing, or other bowel-moving crutches – and also experience few other digestive troubles such as IBS, stomach bloating after meals, excessive gas production, heartburn…

7.   You should urinate roughly once every four hours during the day and NONE at night, always with a consistent yellow color to it (no clear or pale urinations or strong sudden urges).

8.   You should be able to sleep through the night at least 8 hours solid with no wakeups.

9.   If you are a female you should have a timely menstrual cycle with normal flow and very few if any symptoms of PMS, cramping, bloating, and other common complications.

10. If you are a male you should have very full erections and good sex drive. Females should also feel pretty frisky and have good vaginal lubrication with strong sexual urges particularly around the time of ovulation.

There are DOZENS more, but you'll drive yourself nuts trying to notice every tiny thing about your body. These are the basic competencies of good physical function that most deserve your attention. If there was an honorable mention it would probably be moist skin – including skin on the hands and lower legs and feet, which so often become dry when metabolism is reduced. Others might include stable blood sugar, mood stability, good strength and muscle tone, and better than average resistance to colds, flu, and other common infections.

If you are failing in many if not all of these areas, I'm here to help guide you back to better function – and yes, the problems you are experiencing probably are, at least in part, due to your diet and health practices. In the process I want to take the attention away from the small details of nutrition (Is it like, organic? Is it raw dude? What's its antioxidant score? How much fiber is in this?), and redirect you to the primary things to focus on if you hope to achieve immediate and substantial benefit in these main areas.

While we could squabble about the fine details of nutrition for all of eternity, with gruesome PubMed pissing contests and all of the other cheap tricks being employed by the health gurus of the universe, those are really afterthoughts to achieving proper function in the basic areas. Get your machine functioning well and let it handle its own problems, for the most part. This is the 21st century and no one is perfectly healthy, especially not those who dedicate their entire lives to being perfectly healthy. We do the best we can and keep our fingers crossed. What matters is that you feel good enough, and function well enough to live the life you want to live with your time here – with your diet and health practices in the background, not the foreground, of your life.

We'll talk about getting you feeling and performing better soon, but first a short section on some major metabolism-crushing mistakes being made in the pursuit of veganism.

Vegan Mistakes

This will come to make more sense soon when we talk about how to adjust your diet, hydration, and lifestyle for better results. For now, here are some of the most major mistakes being commonly made by vegans and a brief explanation on how metabolism is suppressed through these practices. The Frigid Fourteen…

1. **Not consuming adequate calories…** I've already brought this up and it's a biggie. When you start taking away major food groups like dairy products and meats, you are removing some of the most palatable and calorie-dense foods known to man. Likewise, when you remove major players in the overall sensory enjoyment of eating – the yummiest of the yum, interest in eating often wanes. This may be hardly detectable. Because your hunger may drop you may even feel like you are eating MORE than you

used to or more than you should. But you probably aren't. You may very well have reduced your calorie intake significantly without even knowing it. Calories are energy. If you reduce how much energy you are taking in, the body usually adapts by producing energy at a reduced rate – i.e. reduced metabolism.

2. **Becoming overly puritanical about your eating…** Along the exact same lines, progressing from a vegan diet with lots of calorie-dense foods to one of only fresh, whole foods and lots of greens, vegetables, low-calorie fruits, etc. also spontaneously reduces calorie intake. When the diet migrates from an enjoyable one to a diet built solely around eating foods with the highest ratios of nutrients to calories – the crux of Joel Fuhrman's entire dietary religion and widely-publicized food guide, calorie intake usually drops precipitously and a drop in metabolic rate ensues.

3. **Eating too many cruciferous vegetables…** Cruciferous vegetables are full of chemical compounds known as goitrogens. Goitrogens suppress the thyroid and cause a drop in metabolism that is often quite severe – in some cases even life-threatening if taken to extremes. Vegan mainstays like kale and kale juice, collard greens, arugula, watercress, bok choy, cabbage, broccoli, and cauliflower are often

consumed in dramatic overabundance. Cooking helps to reduce the thyroid-interfering properties of cruciferous vegetables, but vegans often make the mistake of eating or consuming the juice of many crucifers raw with a "the more the better" approach. Raw kale seems to be almost a deified food group in and of itself in many vegan circles. Thanks Joel Furhman. Dick.

4. **Eating too many nuts and seeds…** Nuts and seeds contain higher quantities of a fatty acid called linoleic acid (LA) than any other class of foods. When vegans have few choices for unrefined calorie-dense foods rich in protein, nuts often get consumed in absurd quantities. When I was eating a near-vegan diet it was not uncommon for me to shovel a cup of nuts and seeds into my mouth every day, to speak nothing of the amount of peanut butter I engulfed (not a nut, but nutritionally it should be classed as such). Linoleic acid is an omega 6 fatty acid, and the ratio of omega 3 fatty acids to omega 6 fatty acids is becoming much more widely understood to be of grave importance. Nuts and seeds typically have extremely high ratios of omega 6 to omega 3. Peanuts and Brazil nuts have the highest known ratios of omega 6 to omega 3 of any known foods. Avocadoes, which happen to be practically worshipped and over-consumed by many vegans have similar fatty acid

profiles to most nuts and seeds. Regardless of ratios, and regardless of the fact that nuts and seeds are indeed nutritional powerhouses, LA suppresses metabolic rate on many fronts – from increasing estrogen to interfering with thyroid hormone functionality. For more information on the harms of excessive linoleic acid intake, read some of the impeccably-researched articles at www.raypeat.com

5. **Consuming too many vegetable oils...** Oils from soy, corn, peanuts, avocado, canola, grapeseed, cottonseed, sunflower, and other oils used in many vegan households, vegan products, butter substitutes, and elsewhere also contain very high amounts of LA. Even olive oil contains a considerable amount of LA, although far less than that found in other seed and vegetable oils.

6. **Cleansing, fasting, and detoxing...** While you don't have to be a vegan to practice juice fasts, water fasting, various cleanses including the Master Cleanse and others – this does seem to be much more prevalent and trendy amongst vegans and vegetarians. It's probably a mistake for anyone to do too much of this, but the casualties are particularly severe amongst vegans already suffering from reduced calorie and protein consumption. The short-term effects can feel rejuvenating and even downright euphoric, but most

of this is probably attributable to a large rise in catecholamines and glucocorticoids – stress hormones basically, which are secreted in large amounts when the body is in an underfed state. It feels great in the short term, but not so much as time goes on, like amphetamines. Saying that this slows metabolic rate is a laughable understatement.

7.   **Consuming too many watery foods…** Raw fruits, melons, vegetables, watery porridges, breakfast cereal with soy milk, soups, and other water-rich foods have a general metabolism-suppressing effect for two reasons. The first is that consuming a lot of foods with a high water content fills you up on fewer calories. Fewer Calories = Reduced Metabolic Rate. But in addition to that, and even if you are consuming adequate calories, the excess fluid intake itself is enough to suppress core body temperature and resting metabolic rate. Overhydration, while it's not formally documented anywhere that I am aware, is a very obvious metabolism suppressor for those monitoring basic metabolism biofeedback. When excess fluids are consumed and urine gets very clear, there is a strong tendency to see a drop in body temperature of as much as 2 degrees F with noticeably colder hands and feet. Those with a low metabolism have to be even more careful with this as osmoregulation is extremely impaired when metabolism is low, and overhydration

– or "diluting" it should be called, can trigger a drop in metabolism and many nasty acute symptoms such as blurred vision, anxiety, aggression, dizziness, nausea, erratic pulse, and others – just to name a few. Optimizing the ratio of calories to total fluid intake from all food and beverages will be a prime focus of this book.

8. **Drinking too much water, herbal tea, and other fluids**... Ditto #7 pretty much. I find beverages to be particularly problematic because warm teas and coffee are often consumed by those with a low metabolism to get warm – not guided by thirst. Juices, smoothies, and other supposed health elixirs are often consumed – also not guided by thirst, but because of an internal "idea" that consuming them will yield positive health benefits. Sometimes they do. Mostly they do not. If your metabolism is low, antioxidant-rich teas, green drinks, and triple reverse osmosis Kangen Holy water filtered through Ghandi's robes is about the last thing on earth you need more of.

9. **Consuming too little sodium...** Many vegans also, in their health quest, eschew salt. The main reason this is harmful is that sodium is the primary electrolyte in the extracellular fluid. Sodium is wasted when metabolic rate is reduced so its importance is

heightened. Throw overconsumption of fluids from water, green drinks, smoothies, and tons of watery fruits, vegetables, and soups in there with the sodium-restriction and your body fluids, including your blood, become increasingly diluted. This is referred to as hyponatremia or "water intoxication" and has a lot of nasty side effects that many vegans are experiencing on a daily basis with no understanding as to why.

10. **Doing too much exercise…** Many vegans, not just on a moral quest but one of health and longevity, also add ungodly amounts of exercise – particularly endurance exercise, into their mix of metabolism-suppressing health practices. It's a common misconception to think that exercise "raises metabolism" because doing a lot of it requires that you eat more calories. Using more calories by engaging in physical work does not automatically mean there is a rise in RESTING or BASAL metabolism. Quite the contrary, it usually drops – especially the larger the volume of exercise becomes. Vegan author Doug Graham even states in an article of his that pursuing his dietary practices combined with lots of long-distance endurance exercise drops body temperature (the best indicator of resting metabolism) very well. He believes that 93 degrees F is the optimal human body temperature. Only one mammal has a body temperature this low that I am

aware of – the sloth. You know, the animal that is the symbol of speed, strength, vitality, energy, and fertility. Oh wait, I was thinking of Sloth in the movie *The Goonies*. He was badass, especially when he dropped in on the sail of One-Eyed Willy's pirate ship with a knife. Sloths are those ridiculously slow, weak creatures that sleep 14-hours per day or more and have a bowel transit time of 30 days. My bad. In all seriousness though, lots of exercise in an already compromised metabolic situation is major fuel on the fire, or lack of fire I should say. With exercise alone I've been able to take my body temperature below 96 degrees F and experienced much of the typical dysfunction to be expected in that physiological state.

11. **Eating too many raw foods...** The famous – okay, maybe not famous as no normal person has ever heard of it, Giessen study done in Germany on people eating raw food diets found that being underweight and infertile reached greater and greater magnitude the more raw foods a person ate and the longer they had been going at raw foodism. The human digestive tract, like other human functions, has adapted over millennia to be naturally weaker than that of other creatures. Just like the fact that we don't have a pelt to keep us warm or fast legs to run down prey when we clearly possess enough intelligence to stop wasting so much life energy developing in these areas – so too

is our digestive system ill-equipped to eat food in its least digestible state. A 100% raw food diet may be fine for other creatures, but humans struggle to obtain as much energy from raw foods as they do, and typically fare better supplementing with at least some cooked food. Raw foods also deter calorie consumption due to their properties – requires a lot of chewing, not very calorie dense, fibrous, watery, etc. Most of the biological world functions in a "use it or lose it manner." If you don't subject your bones and muscles to gravity, they atrophy. If you artificially inject testosterone, the glands that produce testosterone will shrink – no longer needed. The body doesn't like to waste energy unnecessarily. In humans, after the dawn of cooking and the unquestionable superiority of cooked foods for assimilation of energy (it's true, all animals, even insects, grow faster and multiply better on cooked foods rather than raw foods), our human digestive tracts adapted to anticipate soft, well-cooked, broken down sources of energy-dense nutrition. Reverting to a raw foods diet usually ends up with a person entering into a state of semi-starvation with the accompanying low metabolic rate. Fruits are the best of the raw, vegan foods – but even sweet, raw fruit is not assimilated to the same degree as cooked fruit and other well-cooked foods.

12. **Eating too little protein…** Vegans always get harassed for lack of adequate protein intake. Some of this harassment is warranted and some of it isn't. The ability to use plant proteins for effective building and maintenance is highly variable between individuals. Plant protein is generally inferior in terms of how well it is utilized also, meaning that 20 grams of something like egg white might require you obtaining 60 grams of protein from some plant source to get the equivalent tissue-building effect from that protein. But one thing is certain – if you do not get enough protein, and enough calories to use that protein efficiently, you will pay. Adequate protein is needed to maintain proper clearance of estrogen in the liver for starters – an accumulation of which leads to a noticeable suppression of metabolic rate. While calories are a more important thing to focus on in the protein department – as adequate calorie intake prevents you from "wasting" your protein (being unable to use it anabolically), there's no doubt that many vegans have made a mistake in not eating enough quality protein. But don't be too terrified of failing to obtain adequate protein. The amino acid profiles of many plant proteins are vastly superior to most animal proteins in some categories – namely, plants are usually much lower in methionine, cysteine, and tryptophan. While those aminos may be good for building tissue, tryptophan has many known negative effects,

methionine and cysteine can raise homocysteine levels
(a known risk factor in heart disease), and eating low
levels of methionine has shown in laboratory research
to extend lifespan as much as any known nutritional
intervention. So don't rush down to your butcher
quite yet.

13. **Consuming too many beans, including soy…**
Wait a second! I said that you may have
underconsumed protein as a vegan and now I'm
saying that consuming too many beans and legumes –
arguably the richest protein sources in the plant
kingdom, could have done you in as well! Protein is
certainly somewhat of a Catch-22 as a vegan. Tons of
beans and soy can be pretty tough on the digestive
tract, and in a slow-moving bowel (characteristic of a
reduced metabolism) beans can outright trigger
bacterial overgrowth of the small intestine – the root
cause of most cases of IBS. This in turn can ramp up
estrogen production from the excess bacterial
proliferation, but of course most beans and legumes,
soy especially, contain phytoestrogens as well, which
are best minimized. Anything you can do to lower
your estrogen exposure is probably a good idea in
today's modern world, full of xenoestrogenic
chemicals, estrogenic vegetable oils, and more. Even
the very act of lowering metabolic rate itself lowers
levels of hormones like testosterone and progesterone

that defend the body against estrogen's many negative effects. A few beans and a little tofu and miso from time to time is probably fine, but I know in my vegetarian days I consumed frightening quantities of legumes and soy milk – and did so to the point where my gut was completely unable to eat these foods without extreme gastrointestinal pain and distress. If you are looking for additional protein as a vegetarian, products like Sun Warrior protein (brown rice protein) or other types of rice protein and non-legume-based proteins are much better supplements. Potatoes, because of their high-quality protein profile and ketoacids, which aid in protein synthesis, are another excellent choice in selecting a safe staple food.

14. **Not supplementing with vitamin B-12...** Well everyone pretty much knows this by now, but this mistake is still being frequently committed by vegans who "feel fine" without it, are freaked out by taking nutritional supplements or anything processed in any way, or just don't understand the essentiality of this vitamin and the unlikelihood of maintaining adequate levels of it as a long-term devoted vegan.

The Net Warming Effect

So far things have been pretty straightforward and simple. I will try my best to keep it that way through this lengthy section.

We have arrived at the nitty gritty now folks. We've talked about the problem – suppression of the metabolism. We've also talked about many of the mistakes that lead to the development of that problem. Now we're set to talk about simple tactics to avoid metabolic problems if you are a vegan or considering a vegan diet, as well as the way home if you have effed yourself up.

The primary things to focus on are the items on the metabolic scorecard mentioned earlier. But it's difficult to focus on 10 things at once. In my experience, you'll get the most out of all this by putting your primary focus on body temperature, warmth of your hands and feet, and overall feelings of body heat – and take things one meal and one snack at a time. The objective is to start experiencing what I call the "net warming effect" from food. The goal is to get body temperature up as early in the day as possible, and then try your best to keep yourself radiating heat from your head to the tips of your toes as much of the time as you can.

If you can do that, and keep it up for many weeks and months consistently, the rest should start to fall into place.

Getting metabolic rate maximized and keeping the metabolism elevated is certainly not as easy and simple as I will be making it out to be in this chapter. But there's no point in making this seem complicated, as the basics aren't complicated at all and yield almost universal improvement.

The first major fundamental thing you should be aware of is the simple fact that stress is the great opponent to metabolism. Therefore, everything you are trying to do in terms of raising metabolic rate revolves generally around suppressing the stress side of the nervous system. When stress hormones become elevated, body temperature tends to fall. Hands and feet also tend to become particularly chilly as stress hormones constrict the blood vessels in your extremities, making your fingers, toes, ears, and the tip of your nose exceptionally cold compared to the rest of you.

Stress hormones are also diuretic – making you empty your bladder whether it's full or not. If your metabolism is really low you will have almost certainly experienced bouts of frequent and excessive urination, strong sudden urges to urinate, nighttime urination, and the tendency for your urine to be really pale or clear. This is not good. Urine concentration and frequency will be another simple bodily sign that we can focus on.

So here we go…

The primary thing you need to focus on is NOT a Joel Fuhrman-like health equation. For those who aren't familiar with Joel, he created a health equation that is Health = Nutrients / Calories. In other words, his belief is that you want to get the maximum number of nutrients with the minimum number of calories – thus gravitating to things that have a high ratio of nutrients to calories. Kale, the low-calorie thyroid-suppressing goitrogen tops his list of ideal foods. Nothing against nutrients, but if you are eating a predominantly "healthy," whole foods type of diet with a lot of unrefined foods, it actually takes a focused effort to get enough calories in. Without adequate calories, no amount of nutrients on earth will deliver a good functioning metabolism. And if you are eating plenty of wholesome foods, the nutrients are going to come with the foods you are eating.

The lower your metabolic rate, the more important calories become. A starving person does not need more kale and bok choy and shots of wheatgrass. A starving person needs concentrated sources of energy. Needless to say, we are all unique little snowflakes with unique circumstances. You will have to figure this out for yourself. This is your experiment. The beauty is in being able to assess whether you are getting the desired effect from the food you are eating, and the lifestyle you are living. But don't be afraid of calories. Celebrate them. Calories are energy, and you can't live at your peak taking in small amounts of energy. And you, if you are experiencing many of the low metabolism signs, may need a breathtakingly large amount of calories to restore your metabolism to its peak.

So, sorry Joel. We're forging a new health equation here. The metabolism equation. The ability of any given meal to stimulate metabolism properly depends on the following…

$$\text{Metabolism Increase} = (\text{Calories} + \text{carbohydrates} + \text{salt}) / \text{Volume} + \text{water content}$$

Thus, you want to select foods, and compose your meals of a high ratio of calories, carbohydrates, and salt in proportion to the volume and water content of the food you are eating.

For conceptual purposes, let's look at watermelon. Watermelon, as the name suggests, has an extremely high water content – over 90%. If you were trying to get 1300 calories from watermelon you would have to eat a 10-pound watermelon, taking in over a gallon (4 liters roughly) of water. That's a huge amount of water and of food by volume for such a measly amount of calories and sodium in comparison.

Speaking of salt (sodium specifically), a 10-pound watermelon has just 45mg of sodium. The same volume of healthy body fluid contains 14,250 mg of sodium – literally 316 times saltier than the fluid in watermelon. You can only imagine how much work the body has to do to keep your body fluids from becoming lethally diluted by consuming this much low-salt fluid. We'll discuss this in more detail later, as it is of extreme importance in this equation.

Let's look at this another way. If you need 1300 calories, by the time you obtained it from a food like watermelon you would vastly exceed your fluid needs, completely dilute the sodium in your body fluids (Our body fluids are salty, like sea water – ever taste tears or sweat? If our fluids aren't salty this causes severe stress and dysfunction to our systems), and never achieve the net warming effect from food. In fact, the more watermelon you eat, the lower your body temperature would likely fall. You can eat it all day long and pee clear all day, feel pretty crappy, even experience very acute negative symptoms attributable to hyponatremia, and be ice cold.

Plus, if you need 1300 calories, who could sit down and consume an entire 10-pound watermelon? Sure, it's been done. But it's not something most people could force themselves to do. Besides, digestion and appetite are often lowered when metabolic rate is suppressed, and it's just not very realistic to think you could get all the calories you need from such a food.

Thus, you need to supplement watery juices, vegetables, greens, salads, soups, water, tea, most fruits, and other foods with a low-calorie density with foods very high in calories – preferably high in carbohydrates and salt as well.

More to come. First, Chris weighs in on his experiences with these small but powerful manipulations…

Chris Randall – Small Changes, Big Results

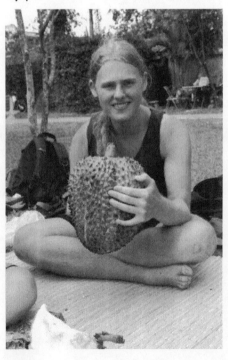

When I very first got onto this whole metabolism/ body temperature thing, it seemed simple enough, yet I had a hard time grasping exactly how to implement it all. It sounded really enticing though. Not having to think for a second, "Am I eating too much?" and eating every single bite of food that I cared for while losing body fat, seeing improvements in strength and performance, better sleep, and actually being able to feel my hands and feet during the winter time? Sounded like a good deal to me.

Before I was used to drinking 2-5 liters of water per day, plus 2-4 coconuts' worth of coconut water, and more watermelon, mangos, cucumbers, tomatoes, absolutely no salt, and very little dried foods. I can't even imagine how much fluid it would add up to in total. Needless to say, I was peeing very frequently and it was always icy clear, rarely even a hint of color. Brrr!!!

All of this was quite a leap for me. I had come from the school of thought that any refined foods (like dried fruit) were sub-optimal, any form of salt was toxic poison, and if you ate any amount of cooked food it meant you just "weren't quite ready" to be all raw yet. Little things kept popping up in my life that stuck out in my head however. I had even heard from several of my fellow 80/10/10 raw vegans that just the smallest of changes, like sprinkling a little sea-salt on their salad in the evenings, left them with a better quality of sleep and a more stable mood.

But who knows? Maybe you feel absolutely fine without any added salt and do your best without it. That's cool. Keep doing what you're doing. But when I see that sprinkling a little salt on their salad keeps a vegan on track and happy with what they're doing vs. running down to the nearest Denny's for 10 orders of chicken wings, I'm going to take note of that.

I'm an open enough person willing to experiment with some things to see if I get different or better results, so I was willing to do a bit of personal testing. How exactly you implement some of these principles into your own diet to get the best results (if that's what you choose to do) will vary greatly from person to person. For me personally, it started out very small. I sprinkled the tiniest bit of Himalayan Salt on top of my salad in the evenings. It tasted amazing and within the next couple of days, I found myself getting significantly better quality sleep, hands and feet much warmer, and overall feeling more relaxed. Before, in my mind logically I knew, "I should be really relaxed and chill right now," but it was like my body didn't want to go with it. This one small change made a massive difference for me.

From there I just thought, "What the hell? I'll just go with it." Before I was comfortable doing what I was doing, but the idea that I could be doing even better and help other people achieve the same was strong for me. I figured I might as well give it a go and jumped into all of the principles you find outlined in this book. Worst-case scenario, I just go back to doing what I was doing before. So I started focusing on balancing out the liquids and caloric density of my diet.

For me, I run my best on lots of sugar, namely from fruit. That was and still is my main staple. What can I say? I like it suh-weet. Nowadays it's a mix of whole fresh fruit, fruit juice, and dried fruit (dates, raisins, dried bananas). A sample meal progression for me might be something like: 1-2 liters of fruit juice, fresh mangos, papaya, or bananas, capped off with something really dense like raisins, dates, or dried bananas. If you can find it, freeze-dried fruit is excellent as well and definitely balances out the juiciness of the fresh fruit. If I feel the need, maybe a little pinch of salt with the dried fruit (It actually tastes excellent) to balance out the previous juiciness.

I drink as much water as necessary, sometimes hardly any at all or up to 2 or more liters if I really need it. Lately I've been enjoying getting much of my fluids from fruit juice as I find it more enjoyable and easier to get in more calories that way. I don't force myself to drink a set amount of water every day like I had in the past. And you know what? I actually feel more properly hydrated from doing so.

See the difference from before, the contrast? Before it was liquid, juicy, and more liquid. Now those components are still there, they are just balanced out by the contrasting denser, drier foods. If you had told me 2 years ago that such a small change in my diet would yield such a big difference in my health, I would have laughed right in your face!

I'll eat some things like potatoes, sweet potatoes, cooked corn, beans/lentils, and rice from time to time now as well. My main focus is fruit, but starches do have a tendency to keep me feeling toasty warm, comfortable and all around feeling great. Things like steamed sweet potatoes with coconut milk/flakes and salt, with maybe some blackstrap molasses and tomato sauce, or white rice with veggies and tamari/soy sauce played a big role in raising my waking body temperatures from a frigid 95.8F to a toasty-warm 97.8-98.2F. If you are someone who's on a strictly raw-food diet and not experiencing the results you'd like, even just a couple baked potatoes now and again might be what it takes to get you back on top.

By the way, if you are someone who wants to maintain a 100% raw diet or feels their best doing so but doesn't want to be so darned cold all the time, I do think you can see massive improvements on a 100% raw diet, slightly tweaked. Including more dried fruit, coconut butter/flakes, not entirely eschewing salt, and not drowning yourself in green juice every single day will definitely de-frost your hands and feet in no time. I still follow a mostly 80/10/10 diet, slightly tweaked. I have some cooked potatoes and beans if and when I feel like them. Minimum of 4,000 calories most days for me.

Seems simple enough though, right? If you're getting down on some juicier foods, follow it up with some drier foods to balance it out. Feeling a bit chilly and peed straight water 3 times in the last hour? Time for something a bit denser and dry with maybe a salty component to it. See? It's way easier than you thought it'd be. How you feel and what exactly you need will change from day to day, but eventually you just get into a groove and things keep pumpin'.

The Net Warming Effect Continued

What I suggest is pretty much ditching low-calorie, watery things almost completely at first until you start warming up considerably. Then, from a healthier and hotter vantage point, you can begin supplementing your diet with more of the iconic juicy "health foods."

Now let's look at a more reasonable example – one of the most calorie-dense fruits, bananas. A large banana contains approximately 120 calories, is very rich in carbohydrates, and is about 75% water. But even with this much more reasonable source of energy, you would still have to eat 10 large bananas to obtain 1200 calories – something few can do without triggering a gag reflex, and in the process of doing so take in an entire quart/liter of water with only a trace of sodium to offset it. For someone with a very high metabolism it might work, but if your metabolism is truly low this is still way too much water and way too little salt to experience the net warming effect. That's why many who try to eat "30 bananas a day" in accordance with the guidelines of the website with that name and preaching such quantities, may still feel cold, flat, and quite ill with metabolism moving in the exact wrong direction.

The only way to make fruits truly "warming" is to cook them (lowering water content), dehydrate them (lowering water content), and/or add concentrated sugar from something like maple syrup or cane sugar and salt. Or you could add fat to increase the calorie-density, turning 5 bananas from a 600-calorie snack into a 1200-calorie feast without increasing the water content at all. Personally I think you'll feel and function significantly better on a diet much higher in carbohydrates than fats though, by percentage of overall calorie intake.

Before we continue with this line of thinking, let's talk about calories. How many calories do you need in a day to increase your metabolism or maintain a high metabolism? Like everything, the answer is "it depends."

In my book *Diet Recovery 2*, a book focused primarily around strategizing for raising metabolic rate, I laid out some formulas for both determining calorie intake for recovery purposes, as well as carbohydrate intake.

While it may not necessarily jive with the relationship you have with eating, I do recommend, especially for vegans with glaringly obvious signs of an impaired metabolism, to become somewhat calorie aware – at least in the beginning. It's important, not to count every calorie to make sure you don't consume too many, but to be generally aware of an estimate of calorie intake to prevent EATING TOO LITTLE. While you may think that the general public is eating too many calories, and that may or may not be true, by far the more common mistake in the vegan world (and health world in general) is eating too few calories, not too many – for all the reasons we've discussed prior. Here is the section from *Diet Recovery 2* on calorie and carbohydrate calculating…

Everyone has their own way of calculating calorie requirements. The main thing to insure success with the objective we're after is making sure that we overshoot your basic needs to achieve metabolism-stimulating surplus. Here's what I have found based on the food reports of others, my own experience, and the common calculations that I've seen used elsewhere…

Because everyone has varying levels of muscle mass, it's best for everyone, as a baseline, to estimate their body weight with very little fat on it. This obviously cannot be precise, but most people have a decent idea of what they feel is their ideal body weight (although when you add a lot of bone mass, muscle mass, organ mass and more during this process you may find you look great, even better than ever before and leaner too at a much higher weight than you expected).

Take this hypothetical, estimated ideal body composition in pounds – let's call it 150 pounds since that is average, and multiply it by 20 if you are a woman and 23 if you are a man.

$$150*20 = 3000$$
$$150*23 = 3450$$

The reason for the difference is that a reasonably lean man and a reasonably lean woman have different body compositions. A man should have more muscle mass and less body fat, and thus have slightly higher metabolic needs than a woman even if scale weight is exactly the same. But, truth be told – and most people know this intuitively, women have higher metabolic rates than men on a lean body weight-adjusted scale. Face it, they are way hotter. No, actually they are. Women tend to have higher peak body temperatures than men – typically coinciding with ovulation and entry to the 2nd half of the menstrual cycle. I actually created a "hot chicks club" for women over 99 degrees F. And, I will add, most women I know can eat just as much as I can despite having way less lean tissue than I have, and my metabolism, while not superhuman, certainly isn't low.

Anyway, those calculations should serve as THE ABSOLUTE MINIMUM amount of calories one should consume on the journey from low metabolic rate to high metabolic rate. With tasty food, it ain't hard. And I wouldn't necessarily back off the calories when body temperature gets up. Rather, I like to see people work on strength and fitness levels while continuing to eat beyond their basal needs.

If you are consuming way more calories than that, great. It's natural if you are coming out of a deficit to see a rapid surge in appetite as you begin "refeeding" as I call it. That big appetite begins to taper as body temperature normalizes. And if it doesn't, that's fine too. The body manages surplus calories very well, increasing the amount passed in stool, increasing physical energy and fidgeting, increasing body heat, and increasing the desire and threshold for exercise. Some people report eating over 8,000 calories per day consistently, without gaining weight, and without going out of their way to forcefully burn calories.

Even a 120-pound woman wrote in the week I'm writing this very paragraph about consistently eating 3500-5000 calories per day and maintaining a rock solid 120-pound bodyweight with no fluctuations.

And yes, if you are over age 30, you will probably consume fewer calories because your metabolism isn't as high as it is in youth, and there is a decline in metabolism with aging that is probably not overturnable (not actually a word, but I think it works). Make sure to eat enough to get that temperature up, but adjust accordingly. If you like calculations, you can probably take your age and subtract 30, then subtract that number from 100 to get a percentage. Then you can multiply that percentage by the calculation above.

So if you are a 50-year old female and your lean body weight is 150 pounds...

$$50-30 = 20$$
$$100-20 = 80\%$$
$$80\% \text{ of } 3000 \text{ calories} = 2,400 \text{ calories}$$

Calculations aside, monitoring basic metabolism biofeedback will show you whether or not you are eating enough to achieve the desired effect. That goes for everybody, young and old.

To determine MINIMUM carbohydrate levels, take your minimum calorie levels calculated above, and divide that number by 8.

For me that's...

$$200*23 = 4600$$
$$4600/8 = 575$$

That 575 is the minimal number of grams of carbohydrates per day needed for optimal recovery, and is equal to about 50% of total caloric intake. But like I said, I would rather see most people slightly tilted to the high-carb side for recovery, and in general, because of the superior properties of sugar and starch for metabolic recovery, and the overall superiority of glucose as a fuel source. 60% carbs might be even better than just half of your energy coming from carbohydrates. Much higher than that though and food becomes too unenjoyable to pack in adequate calories, in my experience. Although you are more than welcome to try it.

Anyway, those are some rough guides for how much to eat to achieve recovery. But like I said in our equation prior, it's not just about calories. If you get all those calories from watermelon it won't make you warm, but increasingly colder. Likewise, if your proportions are structured in a way to achieve the net warming effect, you might get quite warm and feel great despite eating far less than the calculations above dictate.

One example I have used in other materials I have written is the pizza example. Eat a single slice of pizza, which is very high in calories, carbohydrates, and salt – and very low in volume and water, you should get ·

noticeably warmer. However, if you drink a quart of water with that slice of pizza you'll be noticeably cold after.

So the process of stimulating your metabolism probably doesn't require massive calorie intake, but I still think you will feel and function at a much higher level if you err on the side of eating too many calories. I encourage everyone to "EAT THE FOOD" as I always say, in our dieted, calorie-phobic society. And I think it's even more important for vegans, as you really do need to consume quite a few calories to obtain enough protein from low-protein plant foods. If you are to look back at bananas, each one has only about 1 gram of protein, and most need at least 30 grams of protein per day just to keep from wasting away, much less function optimally (most consider, at minimum, that the optimal amount of protein is 1 gram per kg of lean body weight per day).

Okay, now that we've laid down a few basic concepts, let's dig in to what foods to eat, and how to structure meals properly so that you can find that nice, warm zone and be on your way to success.

I have coined what I call the "Anti-Stress S's." While sleep is the mother of all anti-stress activities, often the stress hormones are too active to even get good, metabolism-stimulating sleep. Kinda hard to sleep when your adrenaline is surging (those of you who are accustomed to waking between 2-4 am feeling like you've just had 5 Red Bulls, maybe even having a little anxiety attack and heart palpitations, will certainly be familiar with how hard it is to sleep when adrenaline is peaking... this is the time of day it typically peaks, and the lower the metabolism generally the higher those peaks are).

So we often have to rely on our diet to rescue us from these stress hormones, stimulate the metabolism, and improve our sleep. And the substances most effective at suppressing stress are...

SALT, SUGAR, and STARCH

An honorable mention would be saturated fat. The good news is that the richest sources of saturated fat — coconut and cocoa butter (from chocolate), are both perfectly vegan. And no they won't make you drop dead of a heart attack either. The last time a real researcher thought that to be true I was playing Battleship in Superman briefs and trying to make out with my babysitter's arm... so like, last week is what I'm saying.

When trying to stimulate the metabolism, look at sugar, starch, and salt as a holy trinity that needs to be combined every time you eat. Yes, I'm a HUGE advocate of food-combining. The more foods you combine at your meals the better!

The more you strive to include something sweet, something starchy, and something salty at each meal and snack, the more likely you are to get a substantial rise in metabolism – as long as the foods you choose are calorie-dense enough, and low enough in water content, to keep from exceeding your fluid needs.

I suppose it's time to examine your fluid needs a little more carefully. Then we'll move on to list some specific foods you might incorporate into your diet, followed by some example meals and snacks.

As far as I'm concerned, the world is drowning. Everywhere you look in the modern world people are toting around beverages. The health fanatic totes around big bottles of water or strange fluid concoctions. Meanwhile Jo Schmo is filling up a Big Gulp of Mountain Dew, diet soda, or a bucket-sized coffee thermos. Drink sizes are swelling, and mainstream and alternative health educators alike are preaching to, at the very least, consume 8, 8-ounce glasses of water per day. Some recommend far more.

In reality, these recommendations stem, at the core, from what was discovered to roughly be the average total fluid needs for a person in a 24-hour period. A good rule to go by would be to say that you should shoot for consuming half your body weight in pounds in fluid ounces per day. If you weigh 200 pounds, then this would be 100-ounces of fluid per day, or around 3 quarts/liters. Unfortunately, this somewhat accurate estimate has been twisted to where people think they need to drink this much per day. Not so. That is a better estimate for the total sum of all fluids one should ingest from BOTH food and fluids every 24 hours.

But of course this estimate is limited. The lower your metabolic rate, usually the lower your breathing rate and the lower your skin temperature. These things make your daily fluid needs even lower. Stated another way, the lower your metabolic rate, the less fluid you need to take in. This is yet another reason I suggest that people with a low metabolism eat a lot of foods with a lower water content, while those with a high metabolism can eat a lot more watery stuff. The other reason a person with a low metabolism needs to pay more careful attention to hydrating with the proper amount of fluids, and not excess, is that osmoregulation gets increasingly faulty the lower the metabolism gets as well. In non-geekese, this means that your body is more sensitive to changes in the balance between the ratio of water to electrolytes in your body fluids and cells. It is easier to become dangerously overhydrated, or dangerously dehydrated, when metabolic rate is subpar. A person in perfect health may not need to even give this the slightest thought, but you might – at least until you are functioning closer to your peak.

The estimate for daily fluid intake is also limited because every day is different. One day you eat a really salty stir-fry doused in soy sauce. You will get thirsty and need to drink more to balance that out. Another day you go outdoors in the heat and sweat for 2 hours. Of course you need to drink more that day than others. You really can't give some kind of mass prescription on how to dose your fluid intake to the general public because the need for fluid changes by the hour. Of course, wild animals manage this perfectly without any conscious awareness of what's going on. As humans, we too are hardwired with millennia of evolutionary fine-tuning to keep these systems in balance, if we only listen. It's so fine-tuned that within seconds of something salty hitting your tongue your thirst increases to keep the balance between salt and fluids in your body where they need to be.

Therefore, the only way to really monitor your fluid needs on any given day is to, like anything else, monitor your biofeedback including the concentration and frequency of your urine. I've spent more time paying attention to this than I would care to admit. Everybody says to me, "Dude, urine sane!" Get it, that's um, a joke.

All jokes aside, two peanuts walk into a bar. One was a salted.

I believe that the best ballpark for urine concentration and frequency is to always have some pronounced yellow color to your urine, and urinate roughly every 4 hours during the day and none at night. No stopwatches needed or anything, just a general estimate. If it gets clear, and you are peeing more frequently than that or having particularly strong and sudden urges to empty your bladder, you are overconsuming fluids – or at least consuming too many fluids in proportion to the calories, carbohydrates, and salt you are eating. You remember that metabolism equation thing earlier right?

I hope so, because it's this equation that you use to tweak things in a way that your urine concentration and frequency get in that balanced zone.

Urine clear and happening every 2 hours? Or worse? You urinate and 15-minutes later you feel the urge striking you again? Eat more calories, carbs, and salt and take in fewer fluids. It's not always that simple, but it usually is. You will also note that general body warmth follows the concentration of your urine most of the time. When urine gets clear you will likely feel colder, especially in the hands and feet which are worthy of extra attention. When it's yellow you are more likely to be feeling warm and toasty all over. Remember, the goal is to spend as much time in the warm and toasty all over state as possible. To pretty much live there.

If you do happen to overdo it on the watermelon, or have a lapse in judgment and try to consume nothing but an all-fruit smoothie for breakfast with a glass of water, and you do have an episode of frequent and clear urination – no problem. Just eat…

...A dry, salty, carbohydrate-rich snack or meal as soon as possible.

And lay off the fluids for at least an hour. For convenience-sake I recommend a handful of pretzels or popcorn or some saltine crackers with dried fruit or something, but you're welcome to health-ify it somehow if that makes you feel more comfortable. Have, like, a tamari-dredged hunk of seitan with goji berry sauce – or whatever the hell you weirdos eat. No, I get it. You feel safe that you'll never have your legs amputated if everything you eat is something that your Uncle Diabeetus has never even freakin' heard of.

Okay, you've got that I hope. If not you can read my book *Eat for Heat*, which describes these methods in obscene detail. Yes, it's an entire book, albeit a short one, basically on the above principle alone.

Anyway, here are some of the things I would eat as my staple foods if I were a vegan trying to get my metabolism up. These things are reasonably calorie-dense and perfectly vegan. Next we'll talk about combining things to make meals out of them...

1.   Potatoes – ideally cooked in some coconut oil with plenty of salt
2.   Sweet potatoes and yams – also ideally cooked in a little fat with added salt
3.   Other root vegetables
4.   Rice – well-salted with something like soy sauce would be great

5.   Other grains like quinoa, amaranth, buckwheat, and so on
6.   Dry cereal
7.   Corn – including popcorn, polenta, grits, tortillas, tamales, and all that good stuff – salted
8.   Oatmeal and other porridges – with some added fat, sugar, dried fruit, and salt
9.   Flours – bread, cookies, pasta, pastries, pancakes, waffles, pizza, and other very calorie-dense yummy things made with various grain flours
10. Coconut – coconut oil, coconut milk (not water!), dried coconut, sweetened coconut, coconut ice "cream"
11. Chocolate – cocoa butter, sweetened chocolate, white chocolate
12. Dates – and yummy things made with dates like fruit bars and such
13. Raisins
14. Dried apricots, figs, apples, mango, papaya, and other common dried fruits
15. Sorbets
16. The very sweetest tropical fruits – bananas, papaya, pineapple, mango, cherimoya…
17. Vegan desserts
18. Maple syrup, honey (if you eat it), blackstrap molasses, other concentrated sweeteners
19. Jams, jellies, and preserves
20. Fruit juice (but not too much!)

21. Salted macadamia nuts – pretty much the only nut or seed very low in LA (omega 6)
22. Soy sauce, miso, and other super salty condiments
23. Salt
24. Nutritional yeast
25. Rice protein supplements – like Sun Warrior Protein

Making meals out of these items shouldn't be too hard. I imagine that you are probably somewhere between erotically aroused and scared shitless about some of the foods I just listed above if you've been eating an otherwise puritanical raw food vegan diet or something in the past. Hey, nobody's pressuring you to eat anything. I'm just telling you what will raise your body temperature, and that raising body temperature typically yields substantial health improvements. You do whatever you want.

All you need to do is combine things to be palatable, and make sure that the more watery things you eat, like tropical fruit or fruit juice or floating dry cereal, is combined with foods that offset that water content. You know, the stuff on the left side of the metabolism equation – carbs, calories, and salt. And vice versa. You don't want to eat only dates, dried coconut, and chocolate for a meal and not take in any fluids at all either. It's about balancing the equation, erring on the side of too much salt, sugar, starch, and calories to begin with until you've mastered this.

So let's say you had some pretty watery oatmeal in front of you. If you eat plain oatmeal cooked in water and nothing else you'll be cold and peeing a lot an hour later. However, if you load up the oatmeal with warming elements such as a concentrated source of sugar – something like raisins or maple syrup, a few spoonfuls of coconut milk, and a good pinch of salt… What a difference! No peeing your brains out and you'll be warm for a lot longer before needing to eat again. That's the power of taking something that is watery with very few calories and adding lots of calories and some salt to it without further increasing the water content.

That's how this balancing act is performed.

For lunch, maybe you have a veggie sandwich with some spouts, tomatoes, and a few slices of well-salted avocado. Not bad, but not exactly calorie dense or complete. Have a chocolaty vegan dessert with it and a juicy mango or two. That will probably do the trick and make it a complete meal with something sweet, salty, and starchy with some added fat.

Hopefully you are getting it. Below are some example meals, with beverages included too, that you might be able to see yourself eating throughout the day to keep that body heat pouring out…

Breakfasts:

1.   Oatmeal with dates, maple syrup, coconut milk and salt with 2 bananas
2.   Dry cereal with rice milk, 3 bananas, 3 slices of toast with strawberry jam
3.   Salty potato homefries in coconut oil, glass of orange juice, papaya
4.   Chocolate chip buckwheat pancakes, maple syrup, salted grapefruit
5.   4-banana smoothie with coconut milk, Sun Warrior protein, 2 date muffins

Lunches:

1.   Cous-cous salad with olives, greens, raisins, and macadamia nuts, 1 pound grapes
2.   Hummus sandwich with sprouts, yeast, vegan cookies, glass of juice, 2 mangoes
3.   Salad with mac nuts and raisins, coconut date bars, apple sauce, glass of salted juice
4.   2 mac nut butter and jelly sandwiches, olive oil potato chips, apple, glass of juice
5.   Thai veggie curry, lots of rice, vegan coconut ice cream, fried bananas, tea

Dinners:

1.   Indian potato and pea curry, rice with yeast, Garlic Naan, Mango sorbet, glass of juice

2.   Asian-style stir fry with mac nuts, mushrooms, and veggies with soba noodles, tea

3.   Baked sweet potatoes with shredded coconut, baked cinnamon apples, glass of juice

4.   Mashed garlic potatoes, sautéed spinach, large fruit salad, rice milk

5.   Pasta with tomato sauce, side salad, peach pie, glass of juice

Anyway, that's a small sampling. I'm not saying this is one of those lame "Menu Planners" or whatever brain-dead people like to have. These are just some common foods that may help you envision what your meals might look like. Conceptually, you should be noticing how calorie-dense and salty "warming" foods are in high proportion to the cooling juicy foods like fruit, juice, salads, tea, and so forth.

Your eating can be quite flexible too. Just because I said it's a common mistake for vegans to eat too many beans doesn't mean I'm telling you to strictly avoid beans. Nonsense. Just don't eat them for nearly every meal like I did during a large portion of my vegetarian past. You'll notice that hummus is in one of the meals above, for example. I'm not into strict eating. Not at all. The more strict a person's diet becomes the more at risk they are for developing metabolic problems in my experience, probably because the fewer food options you have the less interesting the food is and the less likely you are to eat enough (or get the anti-stress effect from eating, as this is as much about enjoying your food as it is the calories in them).

Likewise you can customize your own eating to what you like the best, or what makes you feel the best. Some will do better with a lot more starch and salt. Others do great on super sugary diets. Others do best with a relatively even blend of the two.

As your metabolism rises, I would start adding in more and more fresh, juicy foods, and also start drinking some plain water again. Yes, this implies that you probably, as you are first starting out, should drink hardly any water at all. Perhaps not a drop of plain water until your urine has got some color back into it. Just remember to be flexible. What's healing today can be harmful tomorrow. You have to always be attentive to your body and adjust accordingly, free of certain dogmas about what is and isn't healthy. All foods have pros and cons remember? And as your metabolism rises your need for fluids will dramatically increase. I usually drink as much as a full quart/liter of water most days, and more if it's hot or if I'm exercising.

Another important small tip is to add salt where you can. Some need a pretty hefty amount of salt to move towards a high metabolism, especially those who really have a strong desire for salty foods. It may sound strange in places where I wrote "salted juice" or "salted" fruit of some kind. Try it. It's really good. I grew up salting things like grapefruit and grapefruit juice and strongly prefer it over unsalted juice. Lots of people traditionally salt watermelon and things like that too. This is instinctual, just like eating dry, salty, carby snacks when drinking alcohol (something I also recommend if you are going to drink), and it works. Another easy and unexpected place to add a little extra salt is in any of your desserts or baked goods, like muffins or pancakes. And of course salt all the foods that you are accustomed to eating well-salted – like stir-fry or mashed potatoes.

Before we're done here with conversations on food, one important question to ask is "How often should I eat?" In my experience, the lower a person's metabolism, the more often they need to eat. While I listed the basic 3 meals in our examples earlier, in reality most people reading this and in need of undergoing metabolic recovery should eat at least four or five "meals" per day with perhaps some small snacks in addition to that. Obviously if you are breaking your normal 3 meals into 5, each meal will be smaller. That's fine. It's probably best in general to eat small meals frequently instead of big meals infrequently – for everyone. But that's even more important for someone with an impaired metabolism. The higher the metabolism, usually the longer a person can go without food before noticing any negative changes such as feeling shaky, hungry, dizzy, irritable, or cold.

Do the best you can to get to know yourself and the changes you experience when you've gone too long without food. You may notice an hour or two after eating that you start to feel a little chilled, or you get a funky taste in your mouth, or your mood starts to change. That can be a good sign for you to start eating at that interval – be it every four hours or every single hour.

You should also pay attention to the changes in your daily rhythms. You may need to eat more calorie-dense foods in the morning to get warm, and eat more often, but later in the day you can take in a lot more watery food and go longer between meals without crashing and getting cold. That's the typical human rhythm throughout a 24-hour period. Some, however, have almost the exact opposite rhythm. Pay attention and respond accordingly.

And believe it or not, that's it. I wish it was more complex and exotic to better convince you that this was some new medical breakthrough of some kind, but unfortunately it isn't that complex at all. When it comes to playing around with your diet and lifestyle practices, simple and steady rules.

Don't forget sleep and to engage in lots of de-stressing as well as inspirational and creative activities. The more you can rely on those and the less you rely on food to be your metabolism-booster the better. Remember, the battle to keep metabolism high is about beating down stress, and this is rarely done with food alone. Food is just the tool to get you through the doorway and back on your feet again.

Read the FAQ and the Appendix for more important information following some final thoughts by Chris…

Final Thoughts from Chris

At this point, you're probably wondering, "So what the heck is the point of all this? Did this vegan dude experience any benefits from doing this?" From my perspective: absolutely.

The most obvious and notable benefit I've experienced is toasty warm hands and feet and not shivering every moment I'm on an airplane or bus anymore. My unofficial nickname has actually become, "Sweaty Betty." First off, even if I were a chick, my name would certainly not be "Betty." Something a bit more exotic, like "Francesca" or "Zorana." Um, but yes… I am indeed significantly warmer and sweat a heck of a lot more than I used to. So I guess we're halfway there.

Big increases in physical strength, endurance, and muscle growth have been another big plus. My nails (fingers and toes) grow like weeds now too. I swear I clip those buggers at least twice a week. Hair grows even faster and thicker than ever before too. Rock-solid digestion and elimination has been a big note as well. It's like my stomach has turned into an incinerator and I very rarely get any bloating or gas after meals. Going in or out, it's all smooth.

Also, call me crazy, but my beard has been growing more quickly and more fully recently as well. It could entirely be a coincidence with the timing in my life right now (I'm 20 years old as I write this), but I did notice this happening right around the time I saw other things happening with me that were obvious signs of heightened testosterone levels.

Higher sex drive has been obvious as well. I definitely wasn't an asexual prude before by any means, but everything certainly seems to be functioning properly. No oysters or beef liver needed. Waking up "attentively" is the norm just about every day for me now. I'm a firm believer that as a young man, that's definitely one of the signs of a properly functioning body.

Add a massive improvement in quality of sleep to boot, and I've got myself sitting here feeling all warm and fuzzy about the circumstances. I can't seem to ever see those dark circles under my eyes anymore either, even if I'm really pushing it for several days in a row.

So, that's my song I wanted to sing to you, and I hope you enjoyed it.

The big take-away that I want people to get is that if you are experiencing issues on a stereotypical healthy diet, the chances are very slim that being more strict, rigid, and idealistic about your diet and health will result in health improvements. Some of the experiences that I outlined here would have FREAKED me out 3-4 years ago and I would have been absolutely convinced that I was harming myself. My head isn't so big that I can't say that maybe I was wrong about some things in the past, and the information that I have now has the potential to help out a lot of people.

I do see people struggling on 110% raw diets or vegan diets, and I can't turn a blind eye to that. I'm passionate about helping people succeed on a healthy, conscious diet made up of plants. If that means that I have to open my mind and drop the pre-conceived notions I had about certain things before in order to help people succeed now, I'm more than willing to do so. The health of the wonderful people and animals we inhabit this beautiful world with mean much more to me than my ego.

Are you 100% raw? How many grams of fiber do you eat per day? How much green juice do you drink per day? Grams of chlorella powder? Do you ever eat gluten? Pasta???

Frankly, I don't care. What I do care about is that you are a happy, healthy, productive member of this planet and doing your part in making the world a better place.

So go on, have fun. Eat lots of healthy kick-ass vegan food. Move your body in ways that are meaningful to you. Play with your kids. Sing a song. Hell, I'll even forgive you if you play air guitar along to Led Zeppelin IV. Just do something amazing with your life and don't spend all of your day counting up the antioxidant scores or planning how to perfectly combine every bite of food you eat in a day.

Get down and do yo' thang ☺

For more from Chris and how to integrate many of these changes successfully, go to www.realrawresults.com

FAQ

Here are some common questions people have asked me, and that I can envision floating around in your head as you read through this book. This section is not a fluffy unimportant section, but is something that you should read very carefully. There is a lot of information seeded into the responses below that you need to know in advance in order to understand the things you are likely to feel and experience initially as you go about raising your metabolic rate.

Eating all this food makes me feel tired, sluggish, foggy-headed, and bloated. Am I doing something wrong?

Not at all. These are all perfectly normal things to experience as you crossover into a more parasympathetic-dominant state. There are two predominant sides to the nervous system, the sympathetic – synonymous with stress, and the parasympathetic – synonymous with rest, relaxation, growth, and body heat production. A sudden switch from one to the other should feel almost like caffeine withdrawals, making you feel like a lump of sluggish crap. You should really welcome this change though, and look at feeling tired after eating or in general as being similar to being tired after a warm bath or a massage. Relaxing, basically. In my more detailed book about raising metabolism and the recovery process in general I wrote the following...

As you start out, remember that you are challenging your metabolism, your glucose metabolism, your digestion, and more. This does not feel good!!! Headaches, skin breakouts, brain fog, severe drowsiness after meals, out-of-control hunger – particularly if you are coming off of a low-carb diet, heartburn and other digestive glitches – these are all normal in the first week or two. But just when you think you are poisoning yourself with all this food something pretty cool happens. You start to notice improvements in how your body handles everything. Instead of running from all these problem foods and big, heavy meals you experience your body rising to the challenge, making use of the tools you've given it, and functioning much, much better.

So be prepared to be challenged and to have to muster up some resilience and persistence. This is not all fun and games. It's like trying to get back in shape after years of couch surfing. You get tired. You get sore. You ache. But it makes you stronger. You'll see.

I can't tell you exactly what will happen to you as you follow some of these general guidelines. I can't give you timelines on anything either. It all depends. It depends upon your age, your gender, your history, your genetics/constitution, and a lot more that just can't realistically be broken down for each individual. But there are some general things that happen to a large percentage of people when going through this process. I will speak in high percentages, meaning that what I say will happen for most. The peculiar stuff that most people don't seem to experience, I won't delve into. Here goes, starting with the uglier side of things…

Digestive Problems

At first, especially if your diet has been very limited for a long period of time, you will probably collide with some noticeable digestive disturbances. Even switching your dog from one brand of dog food to another is enough to cause digestive upsets for a few days before the digestive tract starts to acclimate to even this simple change. The change you are undergoing may be a heck of a lot more dramatic than switching from Purina to Ol' Roy. So don't let some bowel issues, bloating, acid reflux/indigestion, and other things throw you off course. Expect them, and gear up to be resilient when challenged by them.

Remember, the objective isn't to find the safe foods that keep you from having digestive problems. Take that route and you'll eventually whittle your diet down to practically nothing. Rather, the objective is to improve your digestive abilities, and allow your digestive tract to adjust to eating pretty much anything and everything. This transition does take time. There are even digestive bacteria and enzyme systems that must do a Chinese Fire Drill of sorts for things to start running smoothly. But once this transition is made and your metabolism is ablaze, you should be digesting impossible combinations and quantities of food like a boss. This can take anywhere from a few days to more than a month.

Corpse-like Fatigue

When you go from being in a highly-stressed, underfed state to a de-stressed, overfed state, the adrenal glands pretty much go on vacation. You know how you feel after a big Thanksgiving feast? Your eyelids feel like they weigh a thousand pounds. You feel warm and cozy and tingly all over. All you want to do is pass out into a coma-like slumber. There's a good chance that you will spend a lot of time in this semi-comatose state for many weeks. Maybe even a whole month. If you are recovering from something really severe – like a major eating disorder, this phase can last much longer. Like a whole frickin' year. Don't beat yourself up for feeling utterly unproductive or freak out and think there's something wrong because you're not your former upbeat, energetic self. Spend some time in this state and welcome it openly. It's a healing place to be.

Endocrinologist and author Diana Schwarzbein had a big impact on me with this concept. She states that running on adrenaline and wearing yourself out actually feels really good – whereas rebuilding feels kinda lousy. Like your body and brain have all slowed down by half.

Glucocorticoids, our hormones of stress, can actually create euphoria in large quantities, and shutting them down can cause feelings of near-withdrawal. I have likened eating disorders to a drug dependency, in that eating, once you go beyond a certain point of starvation, actually takes away your internal stimulant meds and makes you feel totally crappy and depressed, with a foggy unfocused brain. Get ready for such feelings, and don't let them fool you into thinking that what you are doing is a disaster.

Menstrual Mayhem

A woman's menstrual cycle is a very sensitive thing. While eventually almost all women notice having more regular rhythms and an absence of all menstrual problems like PMS, water retention, cramping, and so forth – and nearly all women who have lost their periods see it return quickly, very peculiar things can happen to the menstrual cycle for the first few cycles. Chaos is a good word to describe it. It seems that changing the metabolism around represents some big core alterations, and it is not uncommon to have two periods in a month, have an exceptionally heavy or light period or two, pass heinous clots, and have nothing shy of true menstrual mayhem for the first, oh I would say 2-4 cycles after commencing rest and refeeding. As long as you're seeing improvements in many of the other metabolic indicators, don't be thrown off course by this or start seeking out remedies and other diets to "fix" these problems.

Acne/Breakouts

I could design four or five wonderful programs that would make your skin as clear as an anorexic's urine. Zero carb, juice fasts, no-sugar diets – there are plenty. The problem is that most of those approaches, if you are to return to eating everything mixed together like a normal person, will make the skin worse than ever before. If other people can eat everything in sight without having big acne explosions, so can you. It's just a matter of getting your body to function properly.

Well, that's pretty much the pep-talk I give for those worried about re-developing acne when doing the rest and refeeding thing. Some are pleasantly surprised that their acne does not return at all, others do see acne quite aggravated at the start.

If you do notice some breakouts on your face and/or body, expect this to worsen for 1-4 weeks before it stabilizes. Then the skin should become progressively less inflamed until the acne problem clears up and maybe even gets better than it has been in years, with smooth and soft skin. Do not give up on being able to eat all macronutrients and all types of foods with good skin. It is possible to overcome even lifelong tendencies in any area, especially the skin.

Aches and Pains

When refeeding there is often some initial water retention, which can increase physical pain, as well as some pain related to other mechanisms. One of our primary anti-inflammatory internal pain medicines is cortisol. As I mentioned earlier, the adrenal glands that manufacture this cortisol more or less go on vacation. Sometimes there is a transient and temporary period of up to a month or two where pain levels are somewhat higher – especially in joints with a history of aching. Sometimes a small amount of aspirin can work as a reasonably safe pain-reliever.

Changes in Body Composition

When your temperature is below normal, consider yourself primed for some fat gain. From the time temperature is low until the time it reaches the ideal, you are much more likely to gain fat. But it's not all so simple and cut and dry as to think that you will just blimp up doing this. There's a lot more going on underneath the surface.

Before we go any further, it's very important to know, definitively, that our bodies possess an elaborate energy-regulating system. Attempts to consciously override that system usually result in a great deal of backlash, one form being of course a reduced metabolic rate. Another is a reduction in hormones of youth (progesterone, testosterone, DHEA, thyroid, etc.) that have a known tendency to steer ingested food towards the production of muscle tissue, bone, blood, heat, and energy – and an increase in the hormones that favorably steer ingested food towards fat cells (like cortisol).

All the hormones just mentioned are primarily controlled by command central for energy regulation, which is the hypothalamus in the brain. It's not like these hormones act in isolation. But command central doesn't just spin a giant wheel of metabolic fortune to determine how energy should be regulated at random. There are many different factors, a lot of them set into motion before we are even born, such as the number and size of fat cells. The biggest messenger of information regarding energy status comes from hormones like leptin that actually reside in our fat tissue. Pretty novel design actually, as falling body fat levels send a scarcity signal, and rising body fat levels send an abundance signal.

Of course, for reasons not entirely understood by modern science, many a person's hypothalamus is not getting this signal. Regardless of weight or past tendencies or scientific mysteries surrounding "leptin resistance" or any of that, I've found everyone universally responding in the same way to intentional and strategic dietary surplus – the abundance signal is sent. Metabolism rises substantially. Rate of weight gain descends until it stops altogether – usually coinciding with the body temperature reaching "normal."

So, you will probably gain some weight at first, and most of it will be fat and water (the tendency to have edema, or water retention, is much greater the lower the metabolic rate). The weight gained that matters is the fat itself, as hormones in the fat tissue are what send this abundance signal to the brain, in turn rearranging your hormonal landscape to one much more conducive to health and good functioning in all the main body systems (digestive, reproductive, cardiovascular, osmoregulatory, and so on). So don't try to necessarily avoid fat gain. That's like trying to become wealthy by avoiding money. Fat is where it's at.

This fat initially accumulates at a much faster rate around the abdomen than other areas of the body during metabolic recovery. Some think this is due to the body's desire to add fat around the internal organs to protect them from hypothermia (low body temperature). In the past I figured it was to provide an energy supply to the internal organs. It doesn't really matter why. What matters is that it's probably going to happen during the first part of your diet recovery, and that you need to be prepared for it – not freaking out and getting nervous and jumping ship before the next wave of changes.

So, at the start you'll gain weight quickly, then it will slow, and then it will stop altogether. You might only gain weight for two weeks. You might gain weight for several months – maybe 15 pounds the first month, 10 pounds the second, 5 pounds in the third, and then finally none by the fourth month. I recommend just getting the weight gaining part over with. Gaining fat is horrifying. When you stop gaining weight, it's quite a relief and you can focus more on completing your recovery. I call the point of reaching zero fat gain eating enormous quantities of even the most palatable and "fattening" food as becoming "fat-proof." Fat-proofing yourself is a very important first step.

It's also really important to take this process to completion. At first you gain weight around the abdomen, but then you fill out in the rest of your body – adding more subcutaneous fat, which is generally believed to be highly protective and actually healthy. Meanwhile, more and more of your weight gain consists of restored organ mass, bone mass, muscle mass, and glycogen storage. In other words, the LAST 10 pounds you may gain during recovery are the most important pounds. Those pounds restore you to full capacity and also improve how your body looks aesthetically.

Once all of that has taken place, and much of your abdominal fat has been redistributed throughout your entire body, and all your healthy tissue has been restored… THEN, you MAY start losing some body fat. Some do, some don't. But we as humans certainly have the mechanisms that enable the body to shed huge amounts of fat without any conscious effort to cut calories or burn more through exercise. Women after giving birth are a prime example, as they, without any conscious effort, often feel extremely hot and hypermetabolic while shedding 30-40 or even more pounds within the first six months of giving birth. Other women hold onto the weight but lose quite a bit once they stop lactating. It's just a matter of figuring out how to tap into your body's innate ability to do this effortlessly.

I can't, in good conscience, recommend you do anything other than continue to follow the high metabolism and good physical functioning where it leads, and see it through to the end of the cycle – even if it takes several years. I have a feeling, based on my own experience and that of others like personal trainer Billy Craig who has guided dozens of people through the process of high-calorie weight loss, that persistently maintaining a high metabolic rate and eating abundantly on a regular schedule while doing progress-oriented exercise, getting good sleep, and avoiding the yo-yo rollercoaster like the plague, that body fat will eventually come off.

If it does, great. If it doesn't, at least you're healthy and have made a very positive investment in your long-term well-being. One thing is for certain though, no diet or outrageous and unsustainable exercise regimen is going to fix the problem. What that will do is catapult your metabolism right back where it started and re-prime you for more fat gain above and beyond what you would have experienced had you just followed this process to completion. Resist the temptation to diet, and don't get wrapped up in quick weight loss. It will likely come back if you do anything to consciously force it off. In obesity research they refer to that as "intentional weight loss" and it has some nasty after-effects, including contributing to future weight gain past your starting point.

Don't be too nervous though, or let me make you feel like the chances of success are too bleak and that you are forever going to have the body of Mr. Potatohead. They aren't really, and I think you'll find, as many do, that you eventually end up looking more muscular with more prominent fertile characteristics (a more masculine, muscular look for men – a more feminine hourglass figure and shapely look for women, with larger breasts and buttocks).

I started following the general guidelines of this book and immediately started gaining weight – especially right around my belly. I've read that fat around your belly is really bad. Should I stop?

As mentioned earlier, when coming out of a low metabolic state the body will often try to store fat around the internal organs during the first few weeks. Do not be concerned about this – belly fat is the result, not the cause, of stress and poor health. The body is not stupid and committing suicide by storing this abdominal fat. It is a necessary phase of the recovery, and most see it disperse over time as their general health and metabolism have been good for many months consistently.

Once I started doing this I got lots of pimples. What should I change to get my skin clear again?

To reiterate, the objective is not to find the diet that keeps your skin clear, but to have clear skin no matter what you eat. That's a sign of core improvement in the way your body, your inflammatory response, and your detoxification pathways are functioning. Despite the occasional initial worsening of acne, most start to see it improve, and do so continually, after the first month of restoring metabolic rate.

I've been avoiding most starches and sugars because I've been told I have candida. Is it okay for me to eat these foods? Am I just asking for candida to bloom again and cause problems?

When candida is starved it supposedly sends out "roots" or filaments deeper into the digestive tract and beyond. Thus, starving candida can make candida blooms infinitely worse when you return to eating copious quantities of carbohydrates – which most eventually will. When you starve candida of glucose, you also starve yourself of glucose. It's best to nourish yourself well, get good sleep, and optimize your immune system to keep these kinds of things in check. You may experience a profound initial bloom in candida, but this too should resolve itself in due time. Just be persistent and continue to eat lots of the anti-stress, anti-bacterial foods like sugar, salt, and coconut oil in particular.

Sometimes candida is mistaken for bacterial overgrowth of the small intestine, which can cause problems initially as well. As a short-term palliative, until your speed of digestion picks up the pace, raw carrots have natural anti-microbial properties and can help to properly sterilize the small intestine.

I thought nuts and seeds were good for you and had lots of essential fatty acids. If you are not eating them where do you get your essential fatty acids from?

There's probably no such thing as an "essential fatty acid," as the original experiments showing such a thing were probably mistaking nutrient deficiency for the supposed symptoms of a lack of EFA. And if you eat anything containing fat, even fruit, you will obtain such hypothetically "essential" fatty acids. Nuts and seeds probably show a protective effect when studied because they contain lots of minerals, phytonutrients, and vitamin E, which work to counteract the negative effects of the fats in them – and the fats in processed foods containing lots of vegetable oil. But these nutrients can be obtained from other foods without taking in large quantities of linoleic acid.

I have done lots of juice fasts and they made me feel great and helped me lose weight. How can that be bad?

Just because something makes you feel good in the short-term doesn't mean it is good for you. Health would be easy to obtain if we could just do what made us feel good. But unfortunately the body is more complex and needs both active and resting cycles to maintain balance. I believe many of the perceived benefits of fasting and cleanses can be attributed to the large rise in catecholamines and glucocorticoids one experiences when they enter into a highly catabolic state. Inflammation disappears, inflammatory conditions seem to miraculously subside in a matter of days, and so forth. Unfortunately, as one returns to eating normally the inflammatory conditions often worsen over time. The body gets weaker and softer. Digestion slows and weakens. The immune system starts to sputter. Then one continually becomes more and more dependent on fasting to get relief from health problems – each fast providing less relief than the last. It's a vicious cycle that is very destructive to the metabolism in general. I don't recommend getting caught in that trap or overly enamored with the swift anti-inflammatory effects of this unsustainable approach.

There is a lot of information circulating about how bad fructose is for your health. Is it better to eat starchy foods or sugary foods to get your carbohydrates?

I don't think this question can be answered with a purely academic response. Fructose has many properties that make it FAVORABLE to starch. Likewise, starch has some properties that make it favorable over fructose. If I were you I would recommend Freelea (vegan inside joke) consuming both starchy carbs like root vegetables and grains and lots of sugar from fruits, juices, sweeteners, and dried fruit. Then monitor your metabolic biofeedback (temperature, warmth of hands and feet, sleep depth, sex drive, etc.) and determine for yourself what is the best personal fit for you.

Most do best with a combination of starchy foods and sweet foods, if only to decrease the monotony of the diet and thus stimulate greater calorie consumption.

Whatever you do, do not buy into one limited viewpoint you've read in a book, article, or study. Experiment without such psychological baggage knowing that ALL foods have negative and positive attributes, and that certain foods behave a certain way in one context but completely different in another context – some being a better fit for you than others.

Can this work on an 80-10-10 raw vegan diet?

With added salt, extreme favoritism of the more calorie-dense fruits and dried fruits, and a valiant effort to consume copious quantities of calories, it very well might be a suitable diet for sustaining a high metabolic rate. But I think with dietary extremes like this more can go wrong than right. Chris has obviously had some great success with an approach that would classify as 80-10-10, so perhaps he can give you some guidance if you find it not working out as well as you hoped it would.

My temperature is a normal 98.6 degrees F, but I feel cold and have a lot of the symptoms of low metabolism that you describe. Is there any benefit for me to do a refeeding program like this?

Sure. Body temperature is a more reliable metric of metabolic rate than many other easy tests, but it's certainly not foolproof. I have encountered many people with a low metabolic rate and a normal body temperature that responded very well to metabolism-boosting strategies. Focus more on the warmth of the hands and feet and a feeling of greater internal heat production to guide you rather than tracking temperature.

You say that saturated fats don't cause heart disease. I thought it was well-known that saturated fats cause heart disease — and that this was already well-established fact. How can you say otherwise?

There is no such connection. Consider some of the following facts. They should completely confuse you, leaving you feeling like you have no idea what causes heart disease. That's exactly the point. This idea that blood cholesterol is raised by something like saturated fat or cholesterol consumption and that this rise in blood cholesterol has a connection with heart disease is more than just flimsy. It's obviously wrong and much more complex. The saturated fat scare appears to be a perpetuation of a belief that was found to be very lucrative for some rather than something in alignment with modern scientific discovery...

1.   The people with the highest saturated fat consumption, the Masai in Africa have been found to have virtually no heart attacks at any age, with average serum cholesterol levels of 125 mg/dl. When they eat a normal Western diet, much lower in saturated fat, their cholesterol skyrockets.

2.   Blood cholesterol levels increase with age in developed countries. Saturated fat declines with age worldwide, as total calorie intake becomes lower and lower, with total fat and saturated fat intake declining as well. Cholesterol rises, and incidence of virtually all degenerative disease worsens, with a decline in metabolic rate seen with aging, not due to eating too much saturated fat. That is ridiculous. If eating too much saturated fat raises cholesterol, why would eating progressively less of it raise your cholesterol level?

3.   Having low cholesterol is a prominent risk factor for the development of stroke – or having an event that occludes arteries to the brain. The supposed etiology of stroke and heart disease is virtually identical, just involving arteries in different locations in the body.

4.	The more plaque in arteries, the lower the risk for having the most deadly of all known heart attacks – a coronary thrombosis. More plaque equals greater stability and less risk of plaque breaking loose, forming a clot, and acutely cutting off blood supply to the heart.

5.	Just as many people with normal cholesterol have heart attacks as those with high cholesterol.

6.	The population with the highest rates of heart disease – Australian Aboriginal men, have low cholesterol, stellar blood pressure, great HDL to LDL ratios, and other great-looking diagnostics on paper. Yet the rate of heart disease is astronomically higher for them than virtually everyone on earth.

I could go on like this for pages and pages. Heart disease is more complex than it's made out to be in the media, in drug commercials, and in vegetarian literature. Purge your mind of this simple "artery-clogging saturated fat" idea, which is a comical assault to intelligent thought.

I am allergic to many of the foods you mention in the book. Is it still possible for me to succeed in raising my metabolism somehow without many of the foods you recommend?

If your stress and inflammatory responses are primed due to a low metabolism and other factors, allergies, autoimmune disease, and other problems are the norm. But these issues can disappear extremely fast, often by eating lots of all foods, including the ones you have a poor reaction to. I'm not recommending you consume foods you have a deadly allergic reaction to, but things that give you more minor malaise may very well cease aggravating you when you enter into a superior physiological state. Happens all the time, and many have sent reports in of experiencing this really happening, and sharing their elation of the new food freedom they experience. It's certainly worth a shot.

If you cannot seem to conquer your inflammatory reactions to certain foods, it is still possible to raise metabolism with a more limited diet. But it often takes very aggressive food consumption to overcome the monotony of a diet with few food items on the menu.

Almost everyone in the health world says salt is bad for you. Won't eating more salt raise blood pressure and cause other health problems?

That is very doubtful. Cultures that eat a high salt diet are relatively healthy compared to the rest of the world. More reassuring though is a recent study done on salt excretion in the urine that showed some of the most startling statistics I have ever seen. In fact, it could be said from the study that salt is the single-most protective substance ever discovered, as those who excreted the least salt in urine (which parallels salt intake almost exactly) had a death rate that was 500% higher.

Even very high salt diets rarely cause a rise in blood pressure more than a few points. But of course, like anything else, you shouldn't keep eating your body weight in salt every day if your blood pressure has gone up to dangerously high levels and you suspect it is the culprit somehow. There is certainly no reason to fear it outright though, and be timid about consuming it, especially if you have a natural affinity for salty foods.

What type of exercise, and how much exercise should I be doing for a high metabolism?

To go from a low metabolism to a high metabolism, exercise is best kept to fairly low levels – perhaps some light strength training with low repetitions (like 3-5 reps per set, not getting winded or building up lactic acid), and some light exercise well below the heart rate at which lactic acid starts to form (roughly 180bpm minus your age... in accordance with the Maffetone calculation). Once metabolism is up you can do harder training and more vigorous and challenging physical activity within your capabilities. When you overdo it, your temperature will dramatically plummet, so use your own biofeedback to slowly and steadily move towards having both a high resting metabolic rate and exceptional fitness. Just don't rush it or go at it unsustainably. You don't have to feel like you are working hard to make great improvements, and often you will reach greater fitness and maintain greater fitness long-term if you aren't pushing your limits all along the way.

You seem to celebrate consuming large quantities of calories. But isn't there is a ton of information all unanimously showing that calorie restriction prolongs lifespan?

Calorie-restriction prolongs lifespan in laboratory animals, in a sterile environment, with calorie-restriction beginning at birth, in a number of different species. The reasons that none of this is relevant to real-world living as a human being are vast…

1.   Calorie restriction at birth allows a creature to develop smaller than animals of the same species. The smallest members of all species have a higher mass-specific metabolic rate and noticeably prolonged longevity compared to larger members of the same species – small dogs live longer than big dogs, for example. This seems to be the "key active ingredient" in calorie restriction. When your body is already developed, you will get no such benefit from eating a low-calorie diet, but instead will suppress your metabolism, lower your fertility, worsen your sleep, make yourself more nervous and anxious, and

otherwise impair you in just about every perceivable way.

2.   In real life, calorie-restriction makes you hungry. Being hungry in today's world of unlimited food accessibility makes you more likely to binge on calorie-dense food – a pattern seen amongst the obese, known for having repeated starve and binge cycles. Even if calorie restriction works in lab animals, it doesn't work in real humans so neatly.

3.   Calorie restriction and dieting in general often lead to the development of eating disorders, considered to be the deadliest of all "mental" diseases. These illnesses are rapidly on the rise, shave 25 years off of one's life expectancy, and trigger other forms of physical and emotional debility along with it.

4.   The benefits ascribed to calorie restriction may not have as much to do with calories as people think. When calories are reduced, polyunsaturated fat intake is reduced, and methionine – an amino acid, is reduced as well. Diets that reduce these factors are often as successful in the prolongation of lifespan as reducing total energy intake. Of course, as a vegan or vegetarian, methionine intake is already very low, and reducing polyunsaturated fat intake has been discussed throughout this book.

5.   When calorie intake in adulthood falls, the immune system's potency falls as well. A laboratory is a sterile environment, whereas real life outside of a lab

certainly isn't. There are even many links between chronic infections of various types and degenerative diseases like heart disease, cancer, and many autoimmune diseases. It's foolish to assume that reducing calorie intake in the real world would trigger the same effect seen in lab animals with all the variables that are completely unaccounted for.

This is just a short list of things to consider when looking at calorie restriction as a viable tool for life extension. I have considered all these things and strongly feel that a high energy intake, for overall quality and even quantity of life, is the clear choice.

I used to eat lots of calorie-dense food and salt like you describe and felt awful with lots of health problems. Then I went vegan and had lots of green drinks and smoothies and fresh fruits and no salt and all my health problems went away. I feel great now. Doesn't this disprove what you are saying here?

Not at all. I encourage and empower everyone to experiment freely to discover their own, optimal health practices. Going from a junk food diet to a nutritious diet has other variables to be considered too – like clearing up nutrient deficiencies and other intricate things. I still recommend that you take in abundant nutrition, and you will if you eat in the general manner I describe. I also advocate transitioning to an increasingly nutrient-dense diet as metabolism improves. I even grow pea sprouts on my patio for added nutrition in my own diet. There is definitely a middle ground between being a junkfooditarian and realizing the benefits that can be gained from energy-dense foods. I believe we can have the best of both worlds.

I feel like I'm doing everything right according to your guidelines, but I'm not seeing any improvement. Is it possible that I need to bring meat back into my diet to succeed?

Sure it's possible. Meat, and animal products in general have some unique characteristics that can't be acquired from plants alone. I have several people report to me that they start to notice substantial declines in the performance of their metabolism if they don't eat meat at least a couple times per week. I don't think this has to be defeating or looked at as a failure to be humane or environmentally pure either. There is something inherently spiritual about finding what has been mandated to be your own personal nutritional needs at any given stage of your life, and there's nothing immoral about meeting those needs to the best of your ability – regardless of what form that ingested energy takes. Personally, I think if anything, that deriving your sense of morality from what you put in your mouth is very trivial compared to what you could achieve in life if you weren't so distracted by your food choices. Eat meat, eggs, milk, fish, butter, gelatin, and the like if you need to, and do so in celebration of who you are without remorse.

I hear lots of former vegetarians raving about the Paleo diet. If the vegan diet just doesn't work for me and my body, should I try Paleo instead?

The Paleo movement seems to be primarily founded by vegetarians that didn't fare so well as vegetarians but still really care about their health (and believe that you must eat in some peculiar way to attain it). Eating a lot of animal products is often good medicine to correct imbalances incurred on a long-term vegan diet, and the Paleo diet, while it doesn't have to be meat-heavy, usually is.

But I wouldn't recommend jumping from one extreme restricted diet to another. There are a lot of unnecessary restrictions in the Paleo diet, and the diet is often boring and suppressive to appetite and metabolism over the long haul. I certainly wouldn't recommend going low-carb, despite the initial benefits you may experience. It's a long-term dead end for most who embark on it. I think you'll do better, if you can't sustain a vegan diet healthfully, to simply add in a little cheese and milk at first and maybe a beef or fish

entrée a couple times a week if that still doesn't yield
substantial improvement.

*I tried drinking less water, fruit juice, and other fluids and I am
EXTREMELY thirsty, but I am still peeing clear every hour.
Should I drink more or less?*

The body is incredibly intelligent and rarely
sabotages itself. However, dry mouth is a symptom of
excess fluid consumption and the stress response itself.
If you are peeing clear and peeing frequently and
freezing cold in the hands and feet, odds are you need
to eat more salt, sugar, starch and calories and reduce
your total fluid consumption further. When you do get
into a higher metabolic state and your nervous system
calms down, your mouth should get moist, your tongue
pink and rosy, and you should stop peeing like a dog
marking its territory.

Recommended Reading

This is not a blatant commercial promotion. A couple of my other books go into much greater detail on metabolism than I have gone into here. Instead of writing the same thing twice, it makes more sense to me to have you investigate the books I've already written.

Those books are:

Eat for Heat: The Metabolic Approach to Food and Drink
AND
Diet Recovery 2: Restoring Mind and Mood from Dieting, Weight Loss, Exercise, and Healthy Food

I want you to be well-supported and well-informed, and since you have already put some money into this purchase, here is a $5 discount code that you can use towards those two inexpensive books...

1.   Just go to http://180degreehealth.com/180-degree-health-store

2.   Add the two books to your cart

3.   Enter "vegan" in the discount code box

4.   Press update cart

5.   Proceed through checkout with a $5 reduction in price

Appendix- Checking Body Temperature

As a former Broda Barnes worshiper (he's certainly one of the founding fathers of the metabolism-health connection), I used to recommend taking armpit (axillary) temperature first thing in the morning just like he had his patients do, with a target of 97.8 to 98.2 just like him as well. But I'm all grown up now and have ideas and experience of my own. Take the temperature wherever you want, just be consistent. Good morning-temperature targets are 99 butthole, 98.6 oral, 98.0 armpit. I don't know anything about ears and foreheads and vaginas and stuff. I'm old-school I guess. Later in the day temperatures should rise above that.

Armpits are weird though, so I'm kinda steering people away from that now. Sometimes the left and right armpits are a full degree different. That doesn't scream accuracy to me. So go oral, rectal, or vaginal. Man that's fun to write. Here are the best times to gather useful temperature data...

1. Take one temperature first thing upon waking (good way to track how your resting metabolism is changing in response to your interventions).

2. Take another temperature about a half hour after each meal (helps you determine what time of day you tend to need more calorie-dense food, and also how to structure food and fluids to give them the net-warming effect – as your temperature should always rise in response to food... if it doesn't you're either strung out on adrenaline and crashing – which will go away so stick with it, or your meal has too many fluids in proportion to calories and salt).

3. Take another right before you go to bed (if it crashes right before bed, probably a good idea to regularly eat a tasty snack about a half hour before you go to sleep, like a dish of coconut ice cream and something salty like a few handfuls of popcorn).

Do this for a few days, and then just start taking a morning temperature for a while to make sure it is trending upward. It doesn't move in a straight line. It goes up and down and up and down – but generally you should see it moving in the right direction in a general sense.

Women should know that when you start your menstrual cycle your temperatures will drop by about .5 degrees F. Don't be alarmed by this or discouraged. This is normal. After ovulation, your temperature should jump up and be slightly higher than the ideal temp targets listed above.

To make sure your temperature readings aren't artificially low, I recommend warming up your thermometer in your hand or something warm first. You don't want to stick a cold thermometer somewhere or the thermometer itself will actually lower the temperature of the area you are testing.

Once you have warmed up the thermometer to close to body temperature, put it in the testing orifice, then let it sit for at least a half a minute or longer. Then turn the digital thermometer on (a cheap Vicks digital thermometer is as good as any) and get a reading.

If you catch yourself taking more than just a few temperature readings during the day, or taking your body temperature every single day beyond the first few weeks as you start experimenting with this, you might want to throw away your thermometer. It's a useful tool. It's not a license to become obsessive.

If you find yourself inserting your thermometer in and out of one of your orifices repeatedly and panting, call Chris Randall. He specializes in this kind of thing.

After a month or so you should start to know your body metabolically. You should know what having a perfect temperature feels like and when to eat a little more, when to rest a little more, etc. You shouldn't really need a thermometer anymore other than to just check in every once in a while to see if you've fallen off the deep end.

That is all. Have fun.

Oh wait, one more tip. If you use the thermometer in your butt, don't take an oral reading with it right after, heh heh. Or leave it lying around where your kids might pick it up and check their oral temperatures out of curiosity.

References

Articles and Studies:

Cruciferous Vegetables
http://en.wikipedia.org/wiki/Cruciferous_vegetables

How to Make Isotonic Saline Solution
http://www.ehow.com/how_8144429_make-isotonic-saline-solution.html#page=0

Natural Estrogens
http://raypeat.com/articles/articles/natural-estrogens.shtml

Bananas, Raw
http://nutritiondata.self.com/facts/fruits-and-fruit-juices/1846/2

Salt, Table
http://nutritiondata.self.com/facts/spices-and-herbs/216/2

Watermelon, Raw
http://nutritiondata.self.com/facts/fruits-and-fruit-juices/2072/2

Sun Warrior Protein
http://www.sunwarrior.com/product-info/classic-protein/

What You Can Learn from the Q'Ero Diet
http://renegadehealth.com/blog/2010/07/19/what-you-can-learn-from-the-qero-native-diet

Aflatoxin: Another Reason to Shun Peanuts
http://www.marksdailyapple.com/aflatoxins-or-another-reason-to-shun-peanuts/#axzz2PR1gXv6a

Salicylates in Food
http://www.belpernaturalhealth.co.uk/pdf_docs/SALICYCLATES%20IN%20FOOD.pdf

Oxalates in Spinach
http://www.incrediblesmoothies.com/green-smoothies/oxalates-spinach-oxalic-acid-health-concern/

Omega 6 Content of Common Foods
http://180degreehealth.com/2010/02/omega-6-content-of-common-foods

SIBO – Small Intestine Bacterial Overgrowth
http://www.siboinfo.com/diet.html
Suitable Fats, Unsuitable Fats: Issues in Nutrition
http://raypeat.com/articles/articles/unsuitablefats.shtml

Unsaturated Fatty Acids: Nutritionally Essential or Toxic?
http://raypeat.com/articles/articles/unsaturatedfats.shtml

Unsaturated Vegetable Oils – Toxic
http://raypeat.com/articles/articles/unsaturated-oils.shtml

Coconut Oil
http://raypeat.com/articles/articles/coconut-oil.shtml

Vegetables, etc. Who Defines Food?
http://raypeat.com/articles/articles/vegetables.shtml

Methionine restriction increases blood glutathione and longevity in F344 rats
http://www.ncbi.nlm.nih.gov/pubmed/8001743

Lowered methionine ingestion as responsible for the decrease in rodent
mitochondrial oxidative stress in protein and dietary restriction Possible implications
for humans
http://cat.inist.fr/?aModele=afficheN&cpsidt=20677212

Homocysteine and cardiovascular disease: evidence on causality from a meta-analysis
http://www.ncbi.nlm.nih.gov/pubmed/12446535

Low cholesterol is associated with mortality from stroke, heart disease, and cancer:
the Jichi Medical School Cohort Study
http://www.ncbi.nlm.nih.gov/pubmed/21160131

Half of all Heart Attacks occur in people with normal cholesterol levels
http://beyondhealth.com/CustomPages/articles/TheCholesterolMyth.pdf

Coronary Thrombosis
http://medical-dictionary.thefreedictionary.com/coronary+thrombosis

More Masai
http://wholehealthsource.blogspot.com/2008/06/more-masai.html

Aboriginal Health Issues
http://www.betterhealth.vic.gov.au/bhcv2/bhcpdf.nsf/ByPDF/Aboriginal_health_is
sues/$File/Aboriginal_health_issues.pdf

Body Size, Energy metabolism, and lifespan
http://jeb.biologists.org/content/208/9/1717.full

Association between obesity and reduced body temperature in dogs
http://www.nature.com/ijo/journal/v35/n8/full/ijo2010253a.html
Water: swelling, tension, pain, fatigue, aging
http://raypeat.com/articles/articles/water.shtml

Salt, Energy, Metabolic Rate, and Longevity
http://raypeat.com/articles/articles/salt.shtml

TSH, temperature, pulse rate, and other indicators in hypothyroidism
http://raypeat.com/articles/articles/hypothyroidism.shtml

Diabetes, Dangerous fat, and Protective Sugar
http://www.andrewkimblog.com/2013/03/diabetes-dangerous-fat-and-
protective.html

Thyroid disease and the heart
http://circ.ahajournals.org/content/116/15/1725.full

Death rate lower with higher sodium excretion
http://jama.jamanetwork.com/article.aspx?articleid=899663

The Mysterious Origin of the "8 Glasses of Water a Day" rule
http://www.mindthesciencegap.org/2012/10/22/you-need-to-drink-8-glasses-of-
water-a-day-a-history-lesson/

Ingestive Behavior: Drinking
http://home.epix.net/~tcannon1/Physioweek5.htm

Water Intoxication
http://en.wikipedia.org/wiki/Water_intoxication

Hyponatremia
http://en.wikipedia.org/wiki/Hyponatremia

Small Mammal Metabolic Rates: Effect of Body Mass on Mass-Specific Metabolic
Rateand Whole Animal Metabolic Rate
http://www.franklincollege.edu/pwp/lmonroe/Metabolic%20Rate%20Lab.pdf

It's Time to End the War on Salt
http://www.scientificamerican.com/article.cfm?id=its-time-to-end-the-war-on-salt

Nibbling vs. Gorging: Metabolic Advantages of Increased Meal Frequency
http://www.nejm.org/doi/pdf/10.1056/NEJM198910053211403

Low Energy Availability in Female Athletes
http://emedicine.medscape.com/article/312312-overview

Impact of reduced meal frequency without caloric restriction on glucose regulation in healthy, normal-weight middle-aged men and women
http://www.ncbi.nlm.nih.gov/pubmed/17998028
The Problem with omega 6 fat
http://www.cbass.com/Omega6.htm

Hydration Effects on temperature regulation
http://www.ncbi.nlm.nih.gov/pubmed/9694412

Lifestyle and Health aspects of raw food eaters
http://www.ptat.thaigov.net/contents/PTAT_JOURNAL/V23N1/V23N1-KK.pdf

Balancing the Nervous System
http://180degreehealth.com/2010/09/balancing-the-nervous-system-with-cassandra-damiris

Books:

Atkins, Robert. *Dr. Robert Atkins New Diet Revolution.* Avon Books, Inc.: New York, NY, 1992.

Barnard, Neal. *Dr. Neal Barnard's Program for Reversing Diabetes.* Rodale: New York, NY, 2007.

Barnes, Broda. *Hypothyroidism: The Unsuspecting Illness.* Harper and Row: New York, NY, 1976

Barnes, Broda. *Solved: The Riddle of Heart Attacks.* Robinson Press: Fort Collins, CO, 1976

Barnes, Broda. *Hope for Hypoglycemia.* Robinson Press: Fort Collins, CO, 1978

Chilton, Floyd H. *Inflammation Nation.* Fireside: New York, NY, 2007.

Farris, Russell and Per Marin. *The Potbelly Syndrome*. Basic Health Publications: Laguna Beach, CA, 2006.

Fife, Bruce. *Eat Fat Look Thin*. Healthwise: Colorado Springs, CO, 2002.

Fife, Bruce. *The Coconut Oil Miracle*. Avery: New York, NY, 1999.

Fuhrman, Joel. *Eat to Live*. Little, Brown and Company: New York, NY, 2003.

Graham, Doug. *The 80-10-10 Diet*. FoodnSport Press. 2006.

Kendrick, Malcolm. *The Great Cholesterol Con*. John Blake Publishing, Limited, 2008

Keys, Ancel et al. *The Biology of Human Starvation*. The University of Minnesota Press: Minneapolis, MN, 1950.

Langer, Stpehen E. and James F. Scheer. *Solved: The Riddle of Illness*. McGraw Hill: New York, NY, 2006.

McCully, Kilmer S. *The Homocysteine Revolution*. Keats Publishing: New Canaan, CT, 1997.

Sears, Barry. *Enter the Zone*. Regan Books: New York, NY, 1995.

Sears, Barry. *The Age-Free Zone*. Regan Books: New York, NY, 1999.

Sears, Barry. *The Anti-Inflammation Zone*. Collins: New York, NY, 2005.

Sears, Barry. *Toxic Fat*. Thomas Nelson Inc, 2008.

Selye, Hans. *The Stress of Life*. McGraw-Hill: New York, NY, 1976.

Starr, Mark. *Hypothyroidism Type II*. Mark Starr Trust: Columbia, MO, 2005.

Talbott, Shawn. *The Cortisol Connection*. Hunter House: Alameda, CA, 2007.

Wiley, T.S. *Lights Out: Sleep, Sugar, and Survival*. Pocket Books: New York, NY, 2000.

Wrangham, Richard. *Catching Fire*. Basic Books: New York, NY, 2009.

Audio and Video:

"Depressive Symptoms, omega-6:omega-3 Fatty Acids, and Inflammation in Older Adults"
http://www.psychosomaticmedicine.org/cgi/content/abstract/69/3/217

"Suppressor of Cytokine Signaling-3 (SOCS-3), a Potential Mediator of Interleukin-6-dependent Insulin Resistance in Hepatocytes"
http://www.jbc.org/content/278/16/13740.full.pdf

"Eluv Live Interview with Dr. Ray Peat"
http://eluv.podbean.com/2008/10/10/eluv-live-interview-with-dr-ray-peat/

And of course – way too many vegan videos from Durianrider (Harley Johnstone and Freelea), the Fruitarian (Michael Arnstein), Chris's Real Raw Results Channel, Frederic Patenaude, and countless others.

About the Author

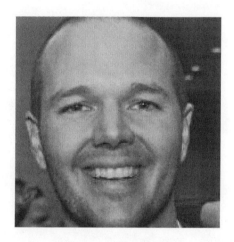

Matt Stone is an independent health researcher and author of more than 10 books on various health-related topics. He launched an independent investigation into health in 2005, and has since been exploring a wide range of health fields - from general physiology and nutrition to areas as diverse and specific as psychoneuroendocrinology. His investigation has yielded many great, practical insights and simple tips on how regular people can make substantial improvements in their health - for the purpose of both improving or eliminating specific health problems and preventing some of the most common ailments in the modern world. Most of his research has drawn him towards metabolic rate and how many basic functions (digestion, reproduction, aging, immunity, inflammation, sleep) perform better when metabolic rate is optimized.

Made in the USA
Lexington, KY
20 December 2013